# THE HISTORY OF THE ACHILLE MARIO DOGLIOTTI COLLEGE OF MEDICINE AND THE LIBERIA POST GRADUATE COLLEGE OF PHYSICIANS AND SURGEONS



ROBERT M. KPOTO, MD

FORTE PUBLISHING

MONROVIA. VIRGINIA. BANGKOK

First Published in 2023 Published by:

**FORTE Publications**
#900 Ashmun Street
Snapper Hill
Monrovia, Liberia
[+231] 88-110-6177

**FORTE Publishing**
7202 Tavenner Lane
# 208 Alexandria
VA, 22306
USA

**FORTE Press**
76 Sarasit Road,
Ban Pong, 70110
Ratchaburi, Thailand
[+66] 85-824-4382

http://fortepublishing.wix.com/fppp
fortepublishing@gmail.com



Printed in the United States of America.

ISBN-13: 978-0-9935710-5-3

# THE HISTORY OF THE ACHILLE MARIO DOGLIOTTI COLLEGE OF MEDICINE AND THE LIBERIA POST GRADUATE COLLEGE OF PHYSICIANS AND SURGEONS

ROBERT M. KPOTO, MD

# Dedication

This book is dedicated to my maternal grandfather, Blama Shello, my maternal grandmother, Kpanah Ngala, my dear mother, Yoko Savo, My father, Noah Sillah (Ziama) Kpoto.

It is also dedicated to all alumni, faculties, and students of both the AM Dogliotti College of Medicine, and the Liberia College of Physicians and Surgeons (LCPS) now and in the future and to the memory of Dr. Samuel G. Bowman, the first Liberian graduate of the Achille Mario Dogliotti College of Medicine (AMDCM).

# Special Dedication

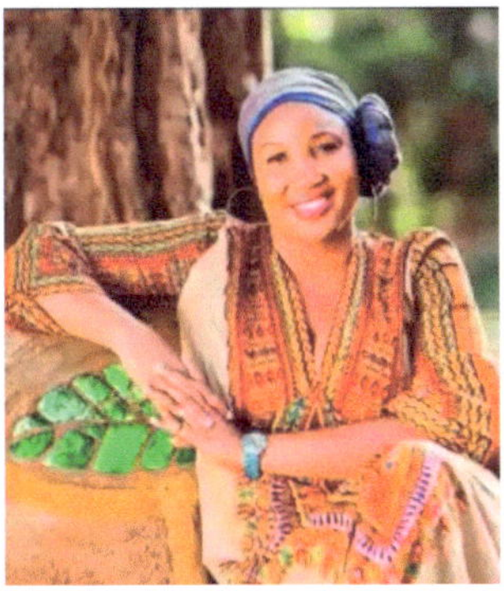

My heartfelt gratitude goes to my dear wife, Dr. Louise Mapleh Kpoto, BSc, MD, MPH (Epidemiology), MMed (OBS/Gyn), PHD Tropical Medicine, who always has and continues to encourage me to unleash my potentials.

She nudged me into telling the story of the pioneers of Achille Mario Dogliotti College of Medicine (AMDCM) and the Liberia College of Physicians and Surgeons (LCPS) as I lived and participated in their geneses.

**ALL PROCEEDS FROM SALES OF THIS BOOK WILL GO INTO A TRUST FUND TO SUPPORT THE RAFA CHILDREN'S SURGICAL HOSPITAL.**

Table of Contents

# Acknowledgement

First and foremost, my thanks go to the Almighty God whose Spirit enlightened me in writing this book.

I would also like to acknowledge my best friend and brother Dr. S. Mohammed Sheriff who always stands by and supports me, pushes, and emboldens me to actualize my true self.

I am specifically indebted to Mrs. Emma Tokpa Miller and Mrs. Klubo K. Zizivily-Cooper both of who spent sleepless nights and sacrificed resting moments to put together this manuscript.

I cannot forget to mention a book that inspired me, titled "**The Purpose Driven Life – What On Earth Am I Here For?**" by Rick Warren. This book helps me to always think beyond the present and to leave a legacy for my purpose on earth into worshipping and serving my **Almighty Creator**, who prepares me for my salvation and has a place in His heavenly Kingdom for me.

Finally, I would like to specifically thank my publisher, Mr. D. Othniel Forte and the FORTE Publishing Company for the editing and ensuring the actualization of this manuscript.

# Foreword

When my friend and brother Professor Robert M. Kpoto asked me to write a foreword to his book "***The History Of The Achille Mario Dogliotti College Of Medicine And The Liberia Post Graduate College Of Physicians And Surgeons*** ", I felt honored and privileged to be a part of this epic legacy.

As a former Deputy Minister of the Ministry of Health and Social Welfare, Chief Medical Officer of the JFK Medical Center Teaching Hospital, as well as former Chairman of the House Committee on Health in the National Legislature I have played a pivotal role in healthcare development and manpower training in the country and therefore I appreciate more the importance and impact of this book.

The book comes 66 years after the visionary President William V.S. Tubman took the first step to achieve his dream of building a medical school as part of his developmental agenda in 1956, and 56 years after the first pre-medical class started at the St. Patrick's School Campus on Capitol Hill in 1966. The journey that began with only 15 students in the first pre-medical class in 1966 has grown to an enrollment of around 239 students per annum as at this writing.

From four graduates of the first cohort, the college has graduated 602 doctors. In like manner, the Postgraduate College which commenced 46 years later with only 19 residents in the first cohort, has trained 110 specialists and now has an enrollment of around 61 students per annum.

Notwithstanding the monumental challenges over the years, the two colleges continue to make significant breakthrough in

Liberia's healthcare services and human resource development.

This book gives a true, firsthand documentary evidence of the colleges' humble beginnings, written by the one who himself was part of that expeditionary journey, along with all those who participated to actualize President Tubman's dream. These pioneers we should cherish and never forget.

Prof. Kpoto chronologically outlines the growth and development of the colleges from their inceptions, and acknowledges those who played cardinal roles at every stage, as well as some of the challenges encountered and successes achieved. He wrote it in short, easy-to-read chapters, with supplementary appendices.

Additionally, some cardinal contents (Rosters of Graduates of each college, the List of Deans, the Hippocratic Oath, the History of the Liberia Medical and Dental Association and the Liberia Medical and Dental Council, the Emblem or Staff, and a Synopsis of Early Torch-bearers) captured in the book qualify it not only as a historical document but also a reference book and inspirational legacy of our noble colleges.

Therefore, without hesitation, I encourage and strongly recommend that every medical student, resident, faculty, library, healthcare training institution, and the public in general, should procure copies of this ground breaking manuscript.

I highly commend Professor Kpoto, who has done a great service to the medical community and the public by producing detailed account of his alma mater in order to serve generations to come.

**_Dr. S. Mohammed Sheriff_**
*Council Member, Examiner and Past V.P. of the*
*West African College of Surgeons*

# Author's Note

My maternal grandfather, Blama Shello, planted in me at a tender age, in our Lofa County Village, Kailahun, the seed of becoming a herbalist and a traditional healer like himself, thus, the code injected in my DNA to become a medical doctor.

My maternal grandmother, Kpanah Ngala, reared me and constantly prayed for me to marry a virtuous wife who would make me happy and help me to be the best version of myself. That answered prayer is embodied in my beloved wife, friend, mother, nurse and advisor, Dr. Louise Mapleh Kpoto.

My dear mother, Yoko Savo, breastfed me till age four and always advised me to be a man and a leader.

My father, Noah Sillah (Ziama) Kpoto, took me from under the comforting wings of my grandfather to send me to school at the age of nine. He convinced me that being a medical doctor was the same as being an herbalist like my grandfather.

# Preface

*"If the lion does not tell his story, the hunter will always be right".*

*African Parable*

I was present through the era of the the construction of, the starting of classes, and subsequently, the graduation of the first (class) cohort from the AM Dogliotti College of Medicine (AMDCM). I have come to realize that most of the younger medical professionals, outside of my generation and the public in general, do not know the history of the AM Dogliotti College of Medicine. This history will not be available for future generations if not told now.

The book specifically explains the true history of both Colleges as I lived, saw, and journeyed through their beginnings. It also highlights the vision of President William V.S. Tubman who established the AM Dogliotti College of Medicine. This information from within me will be irretrievable, if not penned to paper before I transition into eternal glory.

I became more compelled to complete this work when a pioneer classmate and the first Liberian graduate of the AMDCM (AM Dogliotti College of Medicine), Dr. Samuel G. Bowman, transitioned to glory almost INCOGNITO in the medical society.

I therefore pray that, in the years to come, the future generations of these noble colleges, realizing that they have a common heritage, will continue to unite, and remember their pioneers.

Furthermore, it is my prayer that as alumni we continue to make AMDCM a premiere institution of learning for the medical professionals in the sub-region. We should be relentless in providing the needed healthcare that the founding fathers, particularly President William V.S. Tubman, had envisioned for the country.

Robert M. Kpoto

## List of Abbreviations

| | |
|---|---|
| AGSM- | Annual General Scientific Meeting |
| A.M.D. | Achille Mario Dogliotti |
| AMDCM | Achille Mario Dogliotti College of Medicine |
| BSc | Bachelor of Science |
| CMO | Chief Medical Officer |
| CWA | College of West Africa |
| DNA | Deoxyribonucleic Acid |
| Dr. G | Dr. Gwenigali |
| ENT | Ear, Nose & Throat |
| ELWA - | Eternal Love Winning Africa |
| FACS | Fellow of the American College of Surgeons |
| FICS | Fellow of the International College of Surgeons |
| FLCPS | Fellow of the Liberian College of Physicians & Surgeons |
| FRCS- | Fellow of the Royal College of Surgeons |
| FRCSI- | Fellow of the Royal College of Surgeons of Ireland |
| FWACS- | Fellow of the West African College of Surgeons |
| GoL- | Government of Liberia |
| JFK- | John Fitzgerald Kennedy |
| KNUST- | Kwame Nkrumah University of Science & Technology |
| LAMCO- | Liberia American Mining Company |
| LMA- | Liberia Medical Association |
| LMDA- | Liberia Medical & Dental Association |
| LMDC- | Liberia Medical & Dental Council |

| | |
|---|---|
| LCPS- | Liberia College of Physicians and Surgeons |
| LV –PRASAD | Lakkineni (Lakshmi) Vara Prasada |
| MCH (Orth)- | Masters Orthopedic Surgery |
| MD | Medical Doctor |
| MLCPS | Member of Liberia College of Physicians & Surgeons |
| MMED | Master of Medicine |
| MPH | Masters in Public Health |
| NGO | Non-Governmental Organization |
| OBS/GYM | Obstetrics and Gynecology |
| PHD | Doctor of Philosophy |
| SIM | Sudan Interior Mission |
| TNIMA | Tubman National Institute of Medical Arts |
| UK | United Kingdom |
| US/USA | United States of America |
| USAID- | United States Agency for International Development |
| VP | Vice President |
| WHO | World Health Organization |
| WVST | William Vacanarat Shedrach Tubman |

# Section One

The History of Medicine

# Chapter 1

## The History of Medicine

All human societies have medical beliefs that explain birth, diseases treatments, and death. These beliefs are influenced by many factors like culture, tradition, and the beliefs in demons, will of God, taboos, and curses.

The concept of medicine is believed to be as old as creation itself. The Almighty God in His Highness, set the example when He demonstrated the act of Anesthesiology, Surgery and Cloning, according to Genesis 2:21.

It is stated,

"[A]nd the Lord God put Adam to deep sleep", in other words anesthetized him, "[A]nd while Adam was in a deep sleep, He, (God), took one of his ribs out (surgery).

(Genesis 2:22), "[A]nd the rib which the Lord God had taken from Adam, He made (cloning) woman, and "[B]rought her unto man".

This was the first noted biblical example of Anesthesiology surgery and cloning. Man and woman lived happily thereafter until they sinned by disobeying their creator.

They were separated from God and forfeited their immunity from disease, suffering and death. Man, therefore turned to God's creation for answers. He began using herbs and other concoctions to heal his body, and to relieve pain and suffering.

Over subsequent generations the practice has evolved from its crude, trial-and-error forms, to more refined traditional and scientific ones.

Accordingly, in all cultures and major civilizations from Egypt in Africa, to the Mayans and Incas in South America, to Rome and Greece in Europe, and China and India in Asia, we see ample examples of the use of medicine to cure diseases but, it is said that it was not until the time of Hippocrates from Greece that modern medicine is believed to have started.

Hippocrates, therefore, is called the Father of Modern Medicine. He developed the protocol of observation, examination, investigation, and diagnosis and wrote the Great "**Hippocratic Oath**", which is a professional covenant between Doctors and God. (See Appendix 1).

In th e days of the Roman Empire, the emphasis was on hygiene and public health. Their belief was that fitness combats illness. They therefore spent their time becoming fit. That was why the Roman Emperor, Claudius Galen, trained the Roman Soldiers to become fit.

In Greece, Aesculapius, a surgeon, and a pharmacist, developed the present medical emblem, which is also called the Staff. It shows a snake curled around a staff. The serpent was a symbol of health, death, and a messenger between this world and the yonder world.

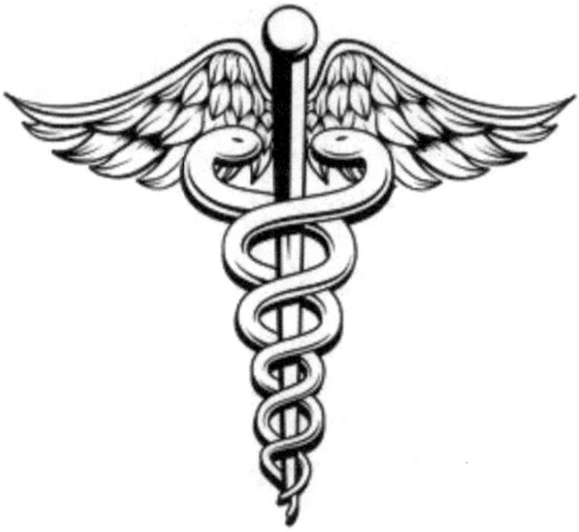

*The Medical Staff*

It was believed that the Almighty God did not intend for man to die. We were, as it may, to shed our skin as the snake does and become new and immortal, continuous living beings.

The other story about the staff is that it depicts the removal of a worm called draconculus meditensis that infests the leg, by slowly curling it around a stick as is shown on the staff.

# Chapter 2

## History Of Medicine in Liberia

As in all parts of the world, medicine is practiced:

(1) traditionally;

(2) spiritually using a constellation of self-made deities from God's creation, particularly creations that are so great beyond human imagination and understanding- e.g., The sun, moon, big mountains, large rivers, dragons, sea, etc. and;

(3) by modern (or western) means.

Traditional and spiritual medicine, still work at home where over a good number of the population in the villages are presently being treated by this method.

Western medical practice was introduced on the west coast of Africa including Liberia by European explorers and colonizers and subsequently by the freed slave settlers and missionaries with whom came medical doctors.

Initially, majority were Caucasians but over time, the *Blacks* trained themselves to become medical doctors, as that would ensure continuity and sustainability for the young nation.

This was necessary because the death toll among white doctors continued to increase and the number willing to come decreased.

Majority of the first group of non-Caucasian doctors were Settlers who trained at Dartmouth University and Columbia College of Surgeons & Physicians in the United States of America.

**In this segment of the book, I highlight specific pioneering Black doctors beginning from the 19th century onwards.**

## 19th Century Pioneers

Although there were many 19th century medical doctors (both Blacks and Caucasians) who pioneered medical services in Liberia, the book focuses on only five (5) Blacks because of their unique pioneering roles in shaping the history of our nation.

Notable among them was Dr. **Samuel Ford McGill.** He was born in Baltimore, Maryland in the US in January, 1815 as a free man. He emigrated to Liberia in 1826 with his family. He returned to the US and graduated from Dartmouth College as a Medical Doctor in 1839. He was the first African-American to earn a medical degree. He returned to Liberia and mentored colonists in medicine for the next decade. Dr. McGill died on June 26, 1871.

***In later years, a group of Liberian consultants at the JFK Medical Center (Dr. Ambrose Wortorson, Dr. Kate Bryant, Dr. Emil Woods) formed the McGill Medical Club (in the early 1970s) in memory of Dr. McGill. The club deserves reactivating.***

**Dr. John Naustedla Lewis** was born in Lower Buchanan, Grand Bassa County in 1845 He was of the Bassa ethnic group from Grand Bassa County, and the first Liberian of indigenous birth to become a medical doctor. He received an M.D. degree from Dartmouth Medical School in early 1873. He settled and practiced successfully in Lower Buchanan for the rest of his life. He passed away on September 2, 1935.

Following him as the second indigenous Liberian to graduate from medical school was **Dr. Henry W. Dennis Hne** (MD 1877) of the Grebo ethnic group from Maryland County.

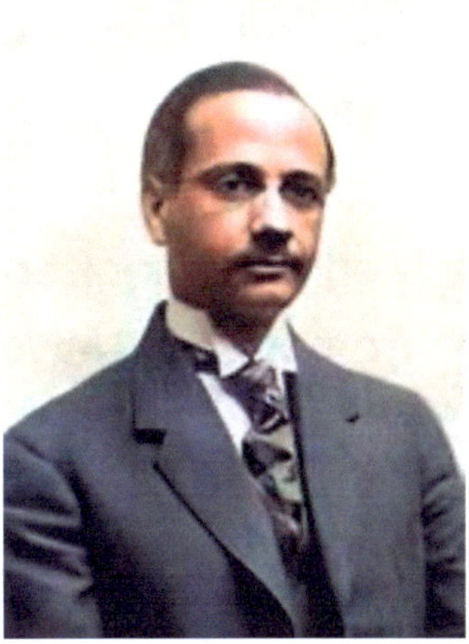

***Solomon Carter Fuller (c. 1911)***
*Psychiatrist*

Outstanding among the early doctors also was **Dr. Solomon Carter Fuller.** He was a pioneering Liberian neurologist, psychiatrist, pathologist, and professor. He was born in Liberia on August 11, 1872.

His paternal grandparents were former slaves that won their freedom and emigrated to Liberia later in their lives. His maternal grandparents were medical missionaries assigned in the colony.

Solomon attended the College Preparatory School of Monrovia. He showed much interest in medicine from an early age.

Fuller then travelled to the USA where he studied at Livingstone College, North Carolina, graduating in 1893. Later he attended Long Island College Medical School. Solomon earned his MD degree from Boston University School of Medicine in 1897.

He pursued further research at the Royal Psychiatric Hospital of the University of Munich, Germany, working with leading researchers like

Emil Kraepelin and Alois Alzheimer.[1]

Dr. Fuller left academia because of racism-disparities in the salary and promotion processes of his time.[2] He continued in private practice as a physician, neurologist, and psychiatrist for many years, until going blind in 1944 and could no longer practice. He died at the age of 81 in Massachusetts.

There is no record of him practicing medicine in Liberia, however, he is known for his work in the field of Alzheimer's disease.

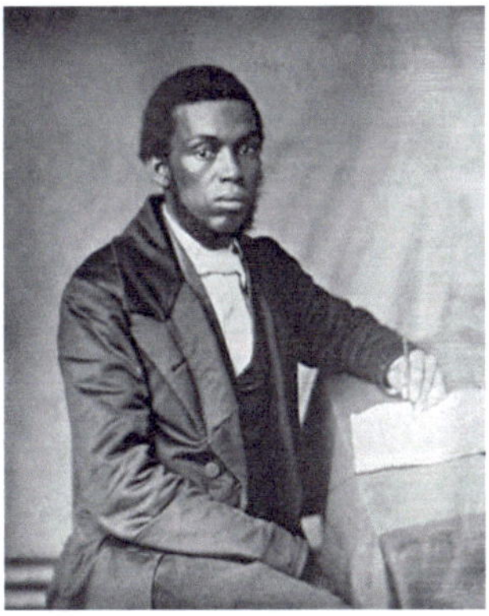

***Dr. James Skirving Smith Sr***
*Physician*

[1] Keith A. P. S., (2008). *A Black Studies Primer: Heroes and Heroines of the African Diaspora,* Hansib Publications, p. 179.

[2] Mohammed, H., (2021). "Recognizing African-American contributions to neurology: The role of Solomon Carter Fuller (1872–1953) in Alzheimer's disease research". *Alzheimer's & Dementia.* **17** (2): 246–250. doi:10.1002/alz.12183. ISSN 1552- 5279. PMC 7986064. PMID 33325137.

Another interesting pioneer medical doctor was Dr. **James Skirving Smith Sr**., the first medical doctor to become president of Liberia.

Dr. Smith was born in Charleston, South Carolina in 1825 and arrived with his family when he was 8 years old. He returned to the US and studied medicine at the University of Vermont College of Medicine.

He obtained his MD in 1848 from Berkshire Medical College in Massachusetts. He returned to Liberia and practiced medicine in Grand Bassa County. He later had a colorful political career beginning in 1856; first as Secretary of State, and later in the 1850s, as Senator of that county.

He became the 8th Vice President in 1870 under President E. J. Roye, and 1871, became the 6th President of Liberia, after President Roye was deposed. Dr. Smith served as President for only two months, from November 1871 to January 1872. He resigned and returned to medical practice and became the Superintendent of Grand Bassa where he passed away in 1892.

# 20th Century Pioneers

Fast-forward to the 20th century, was another famous indigenous pioneer, Dr. **Joseph Nagbe Togba**. Dr. Togba was born on December 18, 1915 in Sasstown. At the age of 17 he was introduced to the practice of medicine and pharmacology at the Nana Kru Methodist Mission by Dr. Everett Veatch, an American missionary physician from Texas. After graduating as class valedictorian at CWA in 1936, Dr. Veatch assisted him in obtaining a scholarship from the Quaker Friends College in Wichita, Kansas.

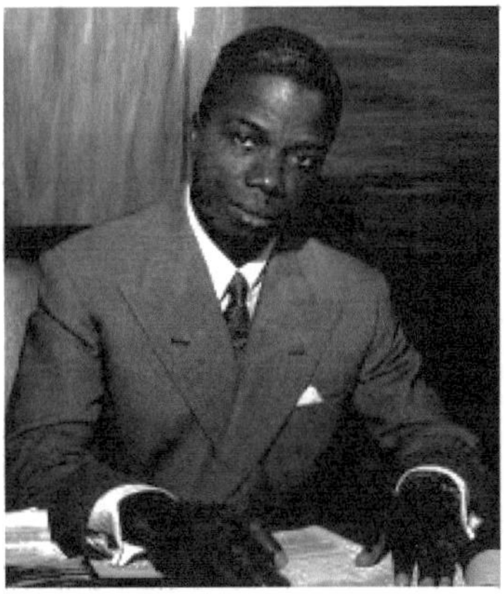

***Dr. Joseph Nagbe Togba***
*Public Health*

He earned his M.D. from the Meharry University in Nashville, Tennessee, United States in 1944. He returned to Liberia where, along with his wife he helped establish the Nursing School, the Liberian Nurses Association, and the Liberian Board of Nurse Examiners. As well as the Liberia Medical Association (LMA) of which he became the first president

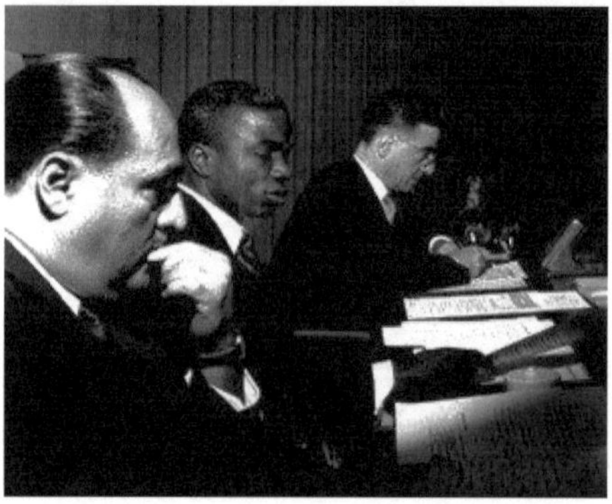

*Dr. Togba at the WHO Charter Signing*

Dr. Togba, considered, **the Father of Public Health in Liberia,** was responsible for setting up the Department of National Public Health Service, now called the Ministry of Health and Social Welfare. He became its first Secretary or Minister. He led the delegation to the founding conference of the World Health Organization in 1948 and was the only black among the original signers of the CHARTER. He died in Silver Spring, Maryland USA on June 13, 2002.

Following Dr. Togba were other indigenous Liberian doctors who took his baton and continued to make significant contributions to health care and man-power capacity building.

***In appreciation of his vast contributions to national healthcare and in particular Public Health, the Liberian chapter of the West African College of Physicians (WACP) conducts an Annual General Scientific Conference in memory of Joseph Nagbe Togba.***

There were other outstanding medical specialist Torch Bearers that followed.

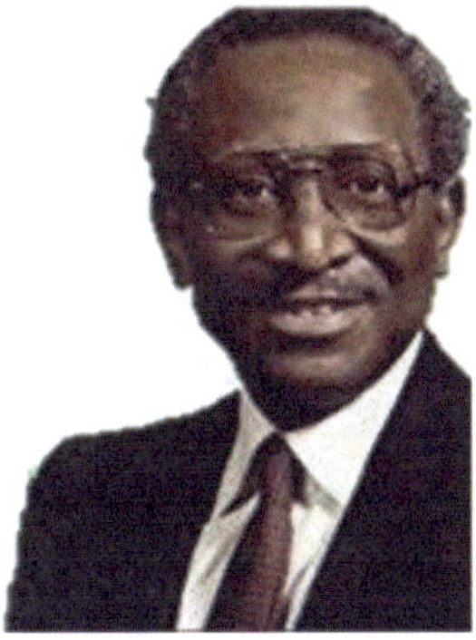

***Dr. Henry Nehemiah Cooper MD, FWACS***
*General Surgeon (Founder Cooper Clinic)*

Dr. Henry Nehemiah Cooper was the first indigenous Liberian surgeon. He was born in the year 1927. He was of the Gola tribe and graduated from the College of West Africa (CWA) in Monrovia. He also studied medicine at Meharry University, like Dr. Togba, graduating with one of the highest scholarship honors.

Young Dr. Cooper returned home to Liberia equipped as the first indigenous specialist general surgeon. He became chief surgeon of the Liberia government hospital. Not long thereafter, when the medical college was established and the JFK Medical Center teaching hospital commenced, he was appointed professor of Surgery and Associate Dean of the College and in addition, Chief Medical Officer (CMO) of the Medical Center.

Dr. Cooper was also the first Liberian to become fellow of the West African College of Surgeons, (WACS). He was a foundation member and subsequently president of the Liberia Medical and Dental Association (LMDA). As a professional medical educator, **he started the first medical outreach program allowing graduands to serve for one year up country after internship.** He is remembered as a brilliant, eloquent, and articulate speaker, a staunch disciplinarian, farsighted and innovative leader, and a worthy role model. Dr. Cooper was also an author. He wrote the authobiographical novel, "The Return of the Guinea Fowl". He passed away at his clinic in 1984 and was buried in Korma.

***In memory of his legacy for the enormous contributions to health manpower capacity development, the Liberian chapter of the West African College of Surgeons (WACS/Liberia) has set aside in April of every year, The Henry Nehemiah Cooper Master Surgeons Memorial Lecture Series.***

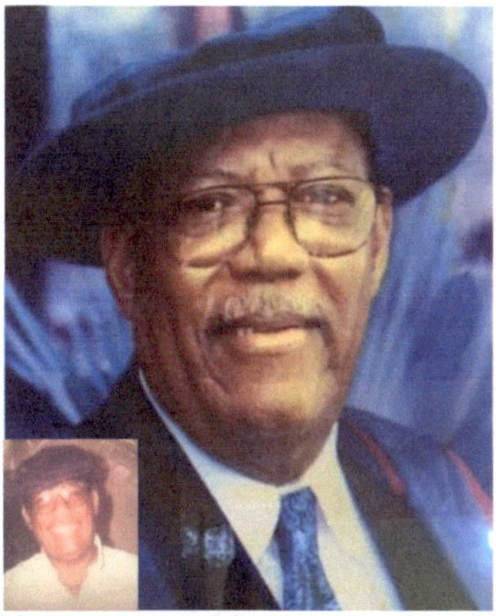

***Prof. Walter Brumskine MD, FRCS, FWACS***
*Urologist*

Professor Walter L. Brumskine was born in 1932. He hailed from Grand Bassa. He obtained his MD from the University of Valencia Medical School in Spain and subsequently England, United Kingdom (UK) where he also studied. He became the first Liberian Specialist Urologist.

Prof. Brumskine was a soft-spoken, brilliant clinician and professor of urology at the A.M. Dogliotti College; contributing immensely to the development of the young minds of Liberian medical professionals.

He was the lone specialist offering urological services to thousands for a very long time. He also served as President Tubman's Private Physician, Associate Dean of A.M. Dogliotti College, President of the LMDA, and an examiner of the West African College of Surgeons (WACS). He passed away on February 12, 2016.

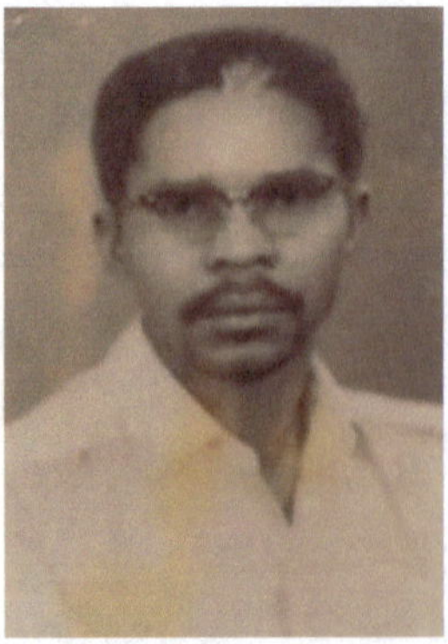

***Dr. Zulu Duma Traub MD, FWACS***
*Ophthalmologist*

Dr. Zulu Duma Traub was a specialist Ophthalmologist. He obtained an MD from Spain and pursued specialization at the Hebrew University of Hadassan in Israel. He was of Kpelle/Gbandi ancestry and was a pioneer of Ophthalmology in Liberia. He was assigned to the Liberian Government Hospital in Monrovia. His litmus test upon his return from studies was to perform a cataract surgery on the nation's President, William V.S. Tubman.

The successful outcome catapulted him professionally in the country. He was quiet but active, humble, down to earth as well as an excellent clinician and teacher.

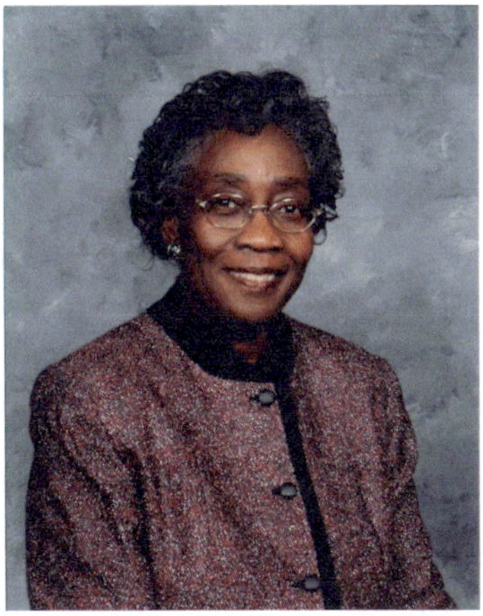

**Dr. Kate Bryant MD, FWACP**
*Pediatric Specialist*

Dr. Kate Bryant is of Vai/Mende root and she hails from Grand Cape Mount County. She is Liberia's pioneer Pediatrician. Dr. Bryant obtained her medical degree in Italy and had additional training at the University of Mekerere in Uganda and subsequently in Britain.

She is a calm, soft spoken, very intelligent and an astute teacher. She headed the Department of Pediatrics at the John F. Kennedy Medical Center until the civil unrest in the 1980s. She also served as a Minister of Health before migrated to the United States.

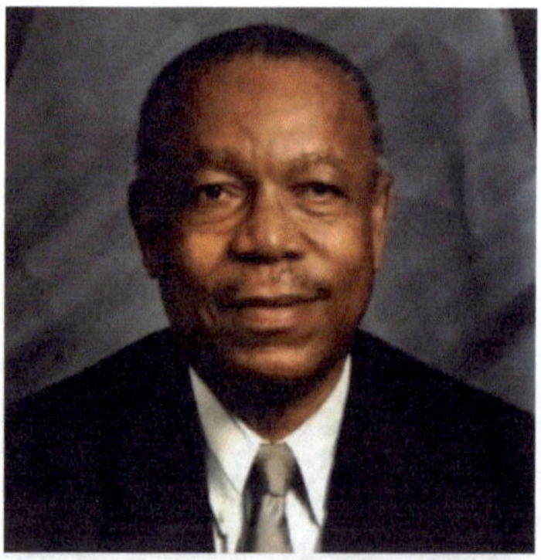

**Dr. Joe Diggs MD, FWACS**
*Radiologist*

Dr. Joe Diggs was a pioneer Liberian Radiologist trained at the University of Switzerland.

He joined the JFK Medical Center, heading the Department of Radiology. Dr. Diggs was an excellent teacher. He left Liberia because of the civil crisis.

### *Dr. Lassana J. Dukuly MD, FACS*

Dr. Lassana J. Dukuly, a pioneer Liberian **Orthopedic Surgeon**, was trained in the United States. He joined the John F. Kennedy Medical Center and worked briefly before the 1980 civil strife that occasioned his departure

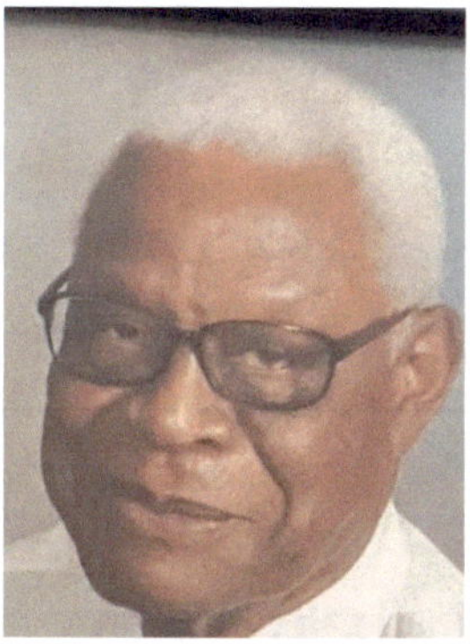

***Dr. Arma Jacob Jones MD***
*Dentist*

Dr. Arma J. Jones was a pioneer Liberian Dentist. He graduated from Sorbonne University in Paris on January 18, 1955. He first worked at the government hospital in Monrovia and later transferred to Harper, Maryland County as the county dentist for several years. Dr. Jones later returned to Monrovia to head the Department of Dentistry at the JFK Medical Center, where he worked until the 1980 coup d'état.

Dr. Jones was a superb dentist and teacher. He was very eloquent in the French language and at times served as French translator for President William V S Tubman.

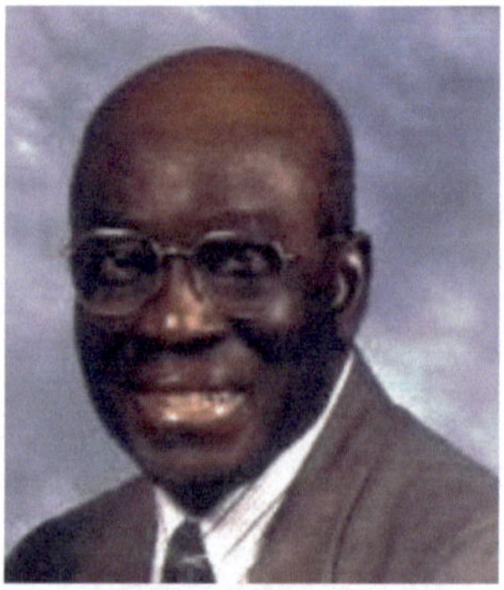

***Dr. Cyril Archibald Johnson MD, FWCS***
*Obstetrician & Gyncologist*

Dr. Cyril Archibald Johnson was born on December 26, 1926 in Monrovia. He was a graduate of the American University of Beirut. He further matriculated at the New York University where he specialized to become an Obstetrician-Gynecologists (Liberia's first).

Dr. Johnson returned to Liberia and was appointed Medical Director of the Maternity Center, and clinical faculty of the A.M. Dogliotti College of Medicine. He was a founding member of LMDA and the Family Planning Association.

He made tremendous contribution to maternal and child care in Liberia delivering over 25,000 babies before he migrated to the United States to escape the civil crisis. Assisting him at the maternity center was Dr. Daniel Collins, MD, who was trained in Spain as the second obstetrician and gynecologist of the era.

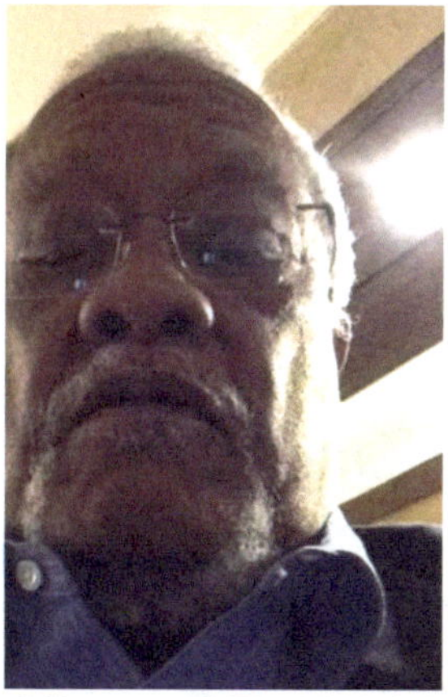

***Dr. Rubel Brewer MD, FWACS***
*Pathologist*

Dr. Rubel Brewer is a pioneer Liberian pathologist trained in Italy. He joined the clinical teaching faculty of the A. M. Dogliotti College of Medicine and was Chief of the Department of Pathology at the John F. Kennedy Medical Center.

During the civil war he left the country and worked with the World Health Organization in the Seychelles.

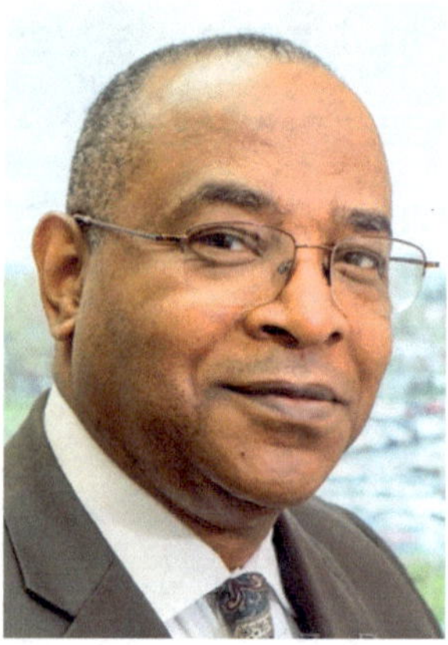

**Dr. Robert Dennis II.**
*Plastic & Reconstructive Surgeon*

Another pioneer Liberian Plastic and Reconstruction Surgeon is Dr. Robert Dennis II. He received his medical degree from Howard University School of Medicine where he ascended to become the head of the Department of Plastic and Reconstructive Surgery.

He made several humanitarian medical relief outreach trips to Liberia to help in the post war health care delivery and rehabilitation process.

Dr. Dennis was eventually persuaded to return

home to take up the posts of Chief Medical Officer at the JFK Medical Center and Associate Dean of the A. M. Dogliotti Medical College. He had a burning desire and passion to reform the Medical Center, but his dream was far in variance with those he worked with, and the government that lacked the political will to facilitate. He cut short his service and returned to the US due to health and family reasons.

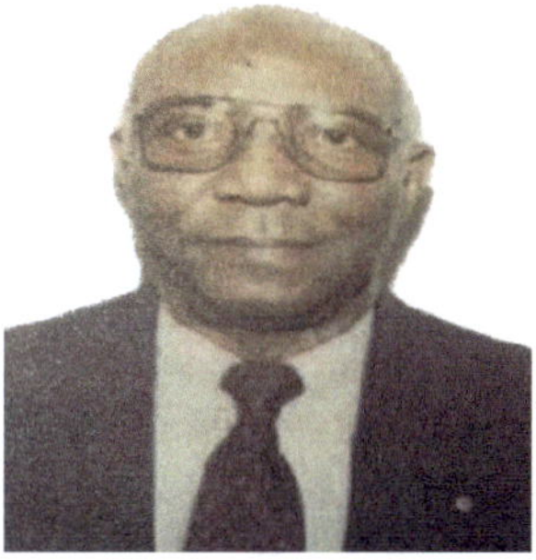

***Dr. Edwin Jallah, MD, FACS, FWACS***
*Cardiothoracic Surgeon*

Dr. Edwin Jallah, with Lorma/Vai roots from Lofa/Cape Mount Counties, was trained in the USA. He was a pioneer Liberian Cardiothoracic Surgeon. Unfortunately, his qualification was far ahead of development at home. As a result, upon his return from training, he ended up working as a general surgeon at the Liberian Government Hospital. Later he was appointed Medical Director at Duside Hospital in Harbel, Firestone where he served until the civil war drove him to the United States.

He was succeeded in later years by **Dr. Jerome Nganana** (FACS), a son of Salayea, Lofa County-as the second cardiothoracic surgeon. Dr. Nganana initially worked at Phebe Hospital with Dr. Gwengale and subsequently transferred to JFK Medical Center to be Chief Medical Officer (CMO) until the civil crisis. Like Dr. Jallah, his cardiothoracic talent was never utilized because of his country's unprepardiness to support him.

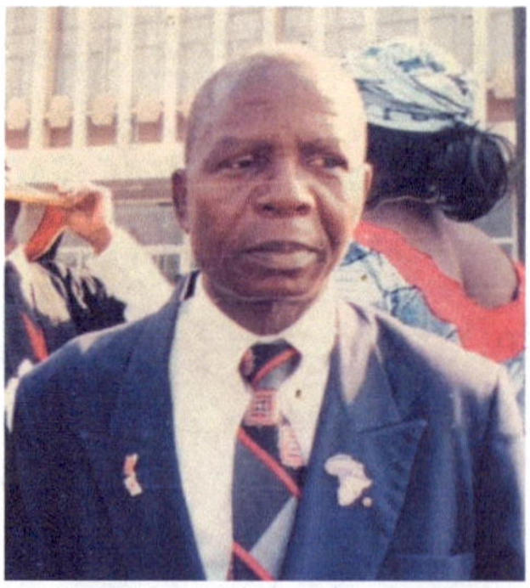

***Dr. Samuel Turwon Dopoe***
*Otorhinolarynologist (ENT)*

Dr. Samuel Turwon Dopoe is a pioneer Liberian Otorhinolaryngologist (ENT) Specialist. Dr. Dopoe is of Gio ancestry from Nimba County. He studied at the University of Bucharest in Romania and later at Charing Cross Teaching Hospital in London.

Upon returning home, Dr. Dopoe joined the faculty of surgery as assistant professor and head of the Department of ENT at the JFK MEDICAL CENTER. He was later appointed Chief Medical Officer/ Deputy Minister, at the Ministry of Health.

During the civil war he was asked to serve as Chief Medical Officer at JFK Medical Center and Associate Dean of the AM Dogliotti Medical College, a position he held until his retirement.

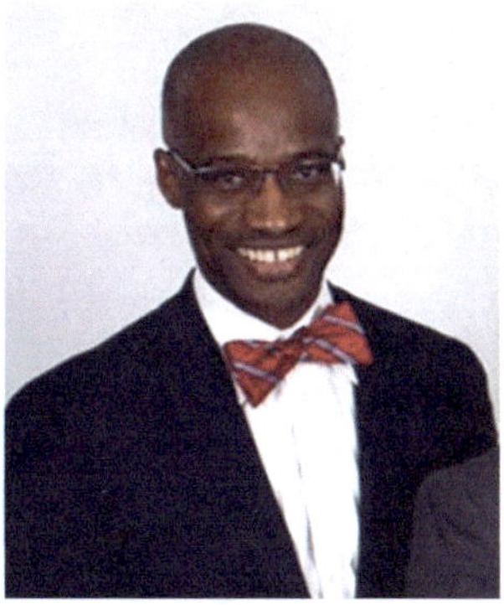

***Dr. Estrada Bernard Jr***
*Neurosurgeon*

Dr. Estrada Bernard Jr. is a pioneer Liberian Neurosurgeon. He studied at Duke University School of Medicine, Durham North Carolina, USA.

He currently affiliates with the Alaska Regional Hospital. His father, ***Estrada Bernard Sr.***, was the former Minister of Health and Social Welfare of the Republic of Liberia, and brother in-law of the first female President of Liberia, Madam Ellen Johnson Sirleaf. Dr. Bernard makes several neurosurgical outreach trips to Liberia from the United States.

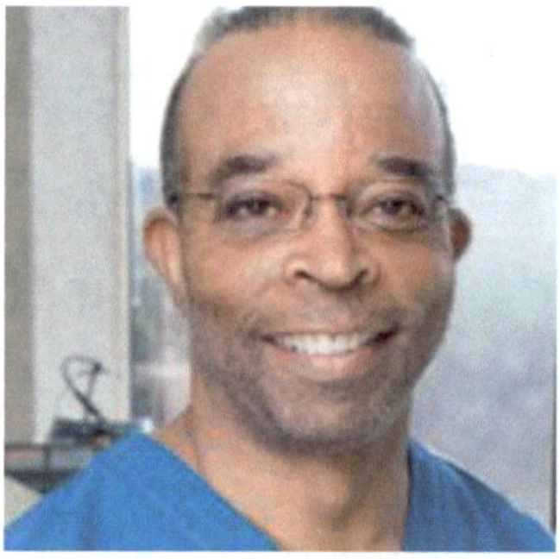

***Dr. Joseph N. Togba, Jr. FACS:***
*Plastic & Reconstructive Surgeon*

Dr. Joseph Togba Jr., is the son of the father of Public Health in Liberia. Dr. Togba Jr. is one of the pioneer Liberian Plastic Surgeons. He trained in the United States.

He returned home and worked briefly as a consultant Plastic Surgeon at the JFK Medical Center but also left because of the civil crisis.

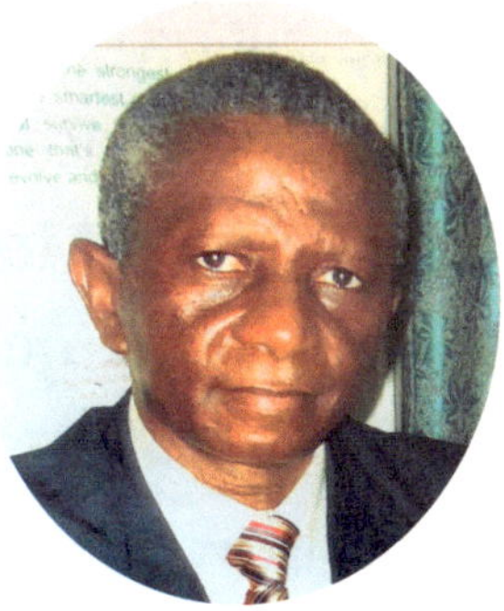

***Prof. Robert M. Kpoto***
*Orthopedic Surgeon & Traumatologist*

A descendant of mixed Lofa tribes (Gola, Lorma, Kissi and Gbandi) Prof. Kpoto was the first Liberian graduate of the A.M. Dogloitti College of Medicine, who through a personal scholarship from President William R. Tolbert, travelled to Britain to pursue advance specialization in Orthopedic Surgery.

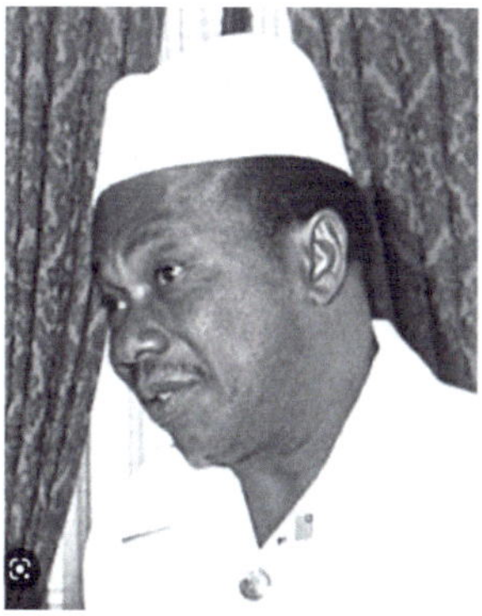

***President William R. Tolbert***

That opportunity supported by documentation, which Prof. Taewor Daramola (Dean) quickly put together, led to the recognition and accreditation of the A.M. Dogliotti College as a medical training institution for the first time by the British Medical Council; thus, paving the way for others to go for postgraduate medical training to the UK.

He obtained fellowship in General Surgery from the University of Dublin in the Republic of Ireland and furthered to the University of Liverpool in England for Masters Degree in Orthopedic Surgery and Traumatology.

Upon returning home Prof. Kpoto joined the Faculty of Surgery and was appointed Head of Department of Orthopedic Surgery at both the J.F.K Medical Center and the Medical College.

For many in the medical profession he is an enviable role model with a deep passion to cultivate young minds and motivate them to pursue advance specialization particularly in the surgical disciplines.

His strong desire to build the human capacity of the healthcare system in the country is unfathomable.

***Dr. Wilmot H Dennis MD, OD***

Dr Dennis was the first Liberian Physician

Physiotherapist. He joined John F. Kennedy Medical Center and was appointed the head of the Department of Physiotherapy. He was also a clinical instructor with the Medical College.

Later, upon the departure of Dean Halay in 1983, he was appointed Acting Dean for the college. He served from 1984 to 1986.

Dr Dennis was a very quiet and reserved individual.

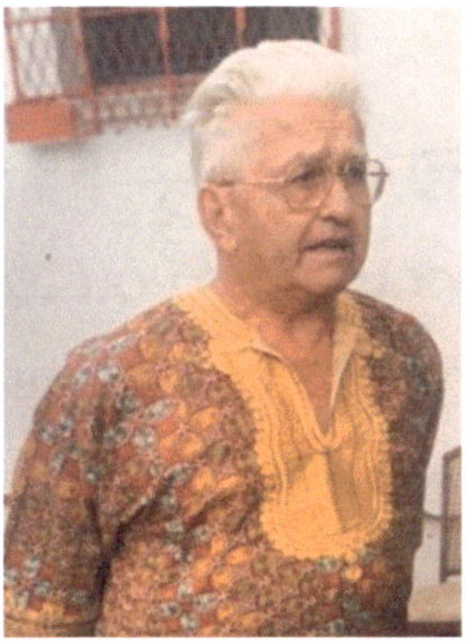

***Dr. Roger J. de Siebenthal***
*Orthopedic Surgeon*

I would like to "bud graft" here with the Liberian Pioneers of doctors, Dr. Roger J. de Siebenthal, the man who inspired and mentored me to become an orthopedic surgeon. Dr. de Siebenthal was a Swiss World War II Air Force Pilot veteran, who came to Liberia as an orthopedic surgeon and traumatologist. He was employed by the Liberia American Mining Company, LAMCO but was eventually recruited by the JFK Medical Center.

He was an excellent surgeon and teacher. Dr. de Siebenthal was very artistic, meticulous, and orderly. He recorded everything he did and was very punctual. He enforced my ambition to be an Orthopedic Surgeon. Upon my return from England, I was appointed head of Department over him; a position I was very reluctant and uncomfortable to accept.

But after consulting him, he said to me, "Robert that is why I encouraged you to study, so that I can give you the *mantle*. Take the position and I will guide you", he advised. And surely, he guided me, not only at the Medical Center but even when I opened my private clinic, he organized my operating theatre and helped to run it. During the civil war, he took care of my mother and sisters in Monrovia, at rebel camp. After the first episode of the crisis, (called World War I), his daughter in Switzerland sent for him. I learned ten years later that he transitioned to glory.

**********

During the early years, health care delivery in Liberia was predominantly the domain of traditional healers, expatriates, missionaries, and concession institutions.

Then, gradually, paramedical training institutions predating our medical college were established by government and missionary institutions to fill the vacuum of the critically needed health care services in the young nation.

Notable among these were:

i. Phebe Nursing School (now Cuttington College Nursing School)
ii. Esther Bacon School of Nursing
iii. Tubman National Institute of Medical Arts (TNIMA) for training nurses, midwives, and physician assistants.

# Chapter 3

## Unveiling A Dream

It is the mid-50s, to be precise 1956, and Liberia is a decade into her development boom. She has a new seaport, Free Port of Monrovia, the largest airport runaway in the sub-region by then, the Roberts International Airport (RIA) and a fancy Capitol Building.

In fact, there are several modern buildings, bridges, and a hydroelectric dam to boast about; not to mention one of the world's fastest growing economies. In furtherance of the growth agenda, President William Vacanarat Shadrach Tubman, the 18th President of the Republic of Liberia, made a state visit to Italy in that year to attract more investments. Whilst in Rome, he paid a call on Pope Pius XII at the Vatican.

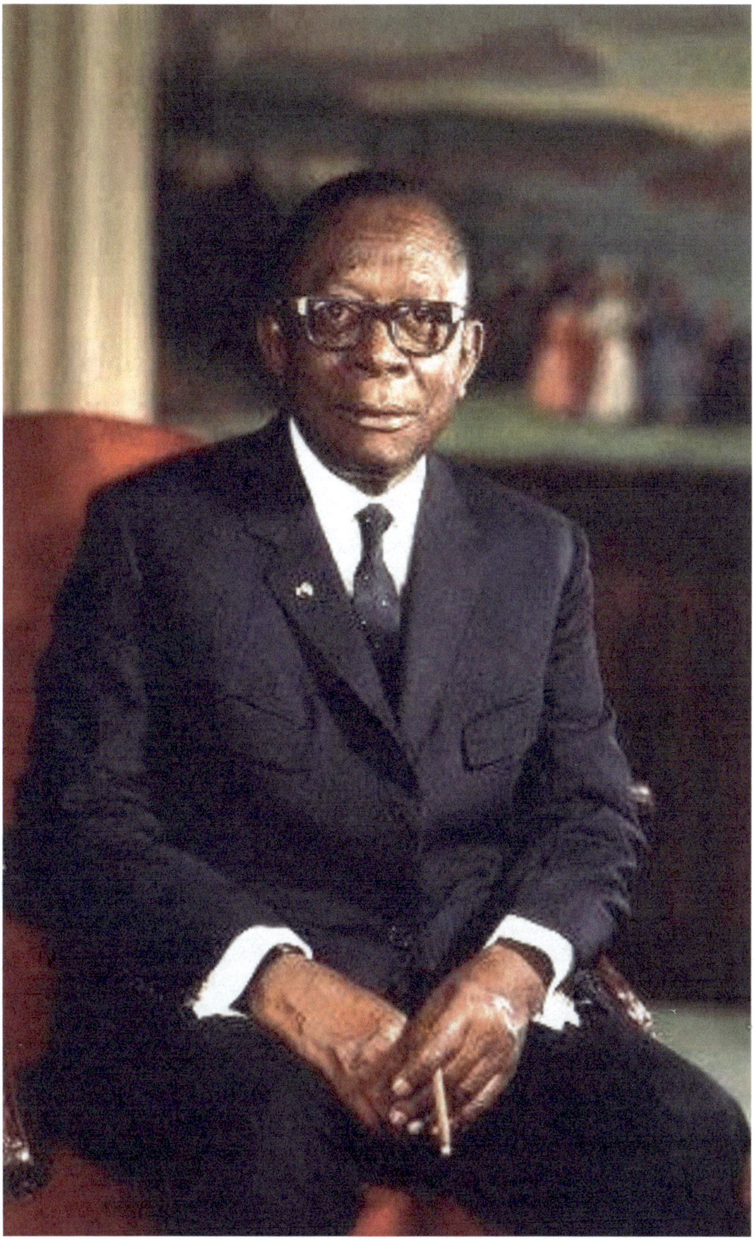

***William V. S. Tubman***
*the 18th President of the Republic of Liberia*

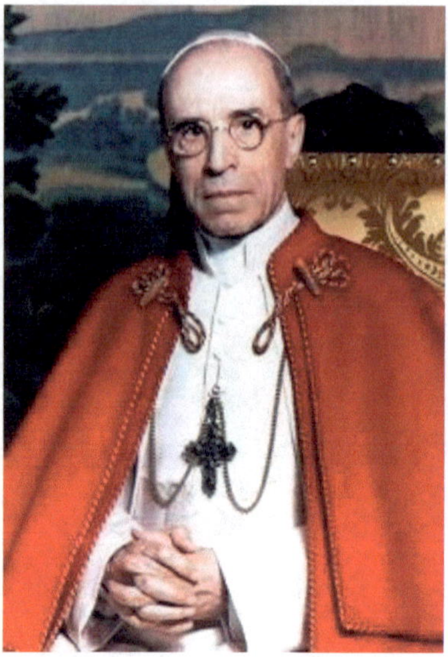

**Pope Pius XII**
*(Courtesy, the Vatican)*

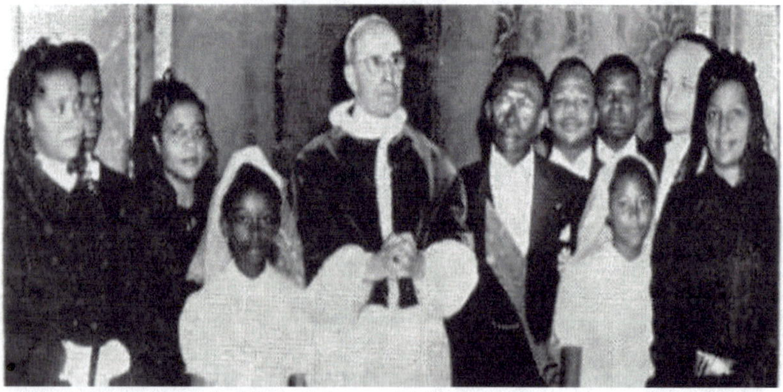

***The Pope and the President:*** *Following a special audience at Castle Gandolfo, Italy, Pope Pius XII poses with Liberian President William V. S. Tubman (left of pope), his wife Antoinette, and daughter Wilhemina (at Pope's right). An official guest of President Giovanni Gronchi, Tubman is reported to have reached agreement for Italian investments in his country. (Courtesy, the Vatican City)*

During the meeting, several aspects of investments and stronger relationships between the two nations were discussed.

President Tubman explained to us (the author and assembly) at the college dedication ceremony, that the Pontiff asked him what he, the Pope, could do to help Liberia? He narrated that his response was spontaneous, precise, and direct. **"I want a Medical College"** as if previously rehearsed.

The President understood that no amount of national development was complete if it did not include a proper healthcare component. The establishment of a teaching hospital and a medical college was important for the nation.

> He vividly remembered the saying **"Give me a fish and I have a meal for a day; but teach me how to fish and I will have meal for life".** In a paraphrase I say, **"Bring me an expatriate doctor, I have health care service for only few years, but train for me a Liberian doctor, I will have healthcare service for life".**

This was the dream the Liberian leader, and all those that followed later had for the establishment of Liberia's first medical college.

By the conclusion of the visit, the parties agreed in principle to establish a medical college and a teaching hospital in Liberia.

The Pontiff then, through the Italian Government, contacted the Dogliotti Foundation of Professor Achille Mario Dogliotti, Rector at the University of Torino, to join and help Liberia open a medical college.

Dogliotti's major task was to ensure the success of the Vatican's commitment to the Liberian government. He would get all the academic resources needed to make that happen.

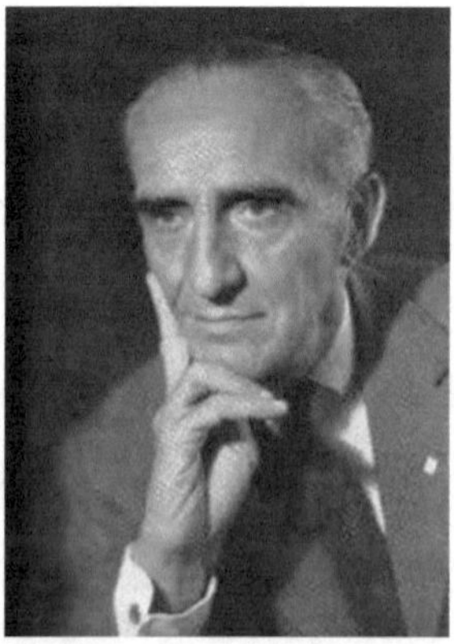

***Prof. Achille Mario Dogliotti***

A further meeting was held in which a tripartite memorandum of understanding was signed between Liberia, Italy, represented by the Dogliotti Foundation, and the Vatican. The roles of the respective members of the triumvirate were very clear:

1. *Liberia, would demonstrate her commitment by giving the land for the construction of the Medical College; protect and facilitate the smooth implementations of the project.*

2. *The Vatican, through the Pope, would cover the cost of the construction of the Medical College and the teaching hospital; and*

3. *The Italian government, through the Dogliotti Foundation, at the University of Torino in Italy, would provide the Professors, the teaching and administrative staff and equipment for the College.*

With this agreement, the parties concluded the discussions and started putting things in motion to fulfill their respective missions.

# Chapter 4

## Rolling Up Sleeves

Upon his return to Liberia, President Tubman began the search for suitable land to accommodate the project. He knew that time was essential if his dream of establishing a medical college would be realized.

He was convinced that this was a priority for his national development agenda.

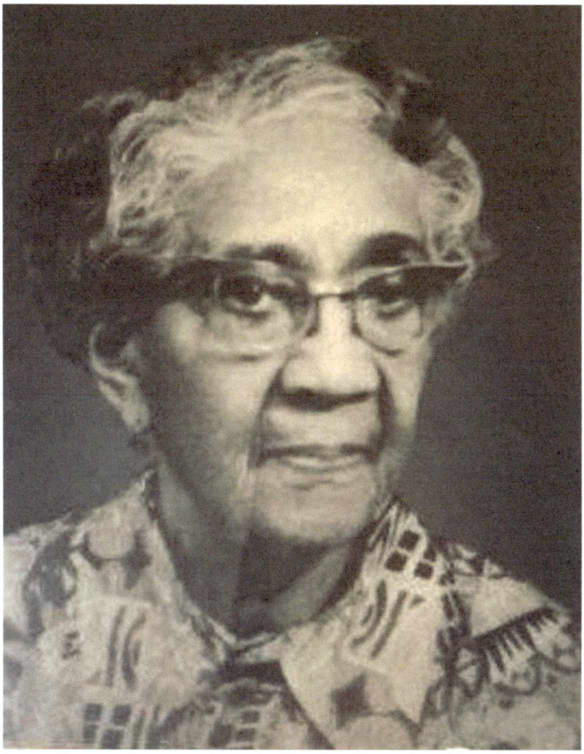

***Martha Eva McGill Hilton (1889-1982)***

By fortune, a Liberian philanthropist, Martha Eva McGill Hilton, probably a descendant of Dr. Samuel Ford McGill, donated **33.5** acres of land in Congo Town, the location now housing the College of Medicine and the St. Joseph's Catholic Hospital.

For almost a decade, 1956 to 1964, meticulous planning by all parties went on- to make available the logistics for the project. And from 1964 to 1966, serious mobilization and implementation commenced.

The University of Torino, located in the City of Torin was the Italian academic institution assigned the task of developing and implementing the curriculum of the medical school.

The parties agreed that the new medical school should be named the **Monrovia- Torino College of Medicine.** It would then be an affiliate of the Faculty of Medicine and Surgery of the University of Torino. The construction of the Monrovia- Torino College of Medicine began in 1966.

The original building plan for the medical school included an academic building, a teaching hospital (currently the St. Joseph's Catholic Hospital), a dormitory and an administrative building.

The initial idea was that the College of Medicine would start its Clinicals on campus using the St. Joseph's Catholic Hospital as the Teaching Hospital. This all looked good on paper.

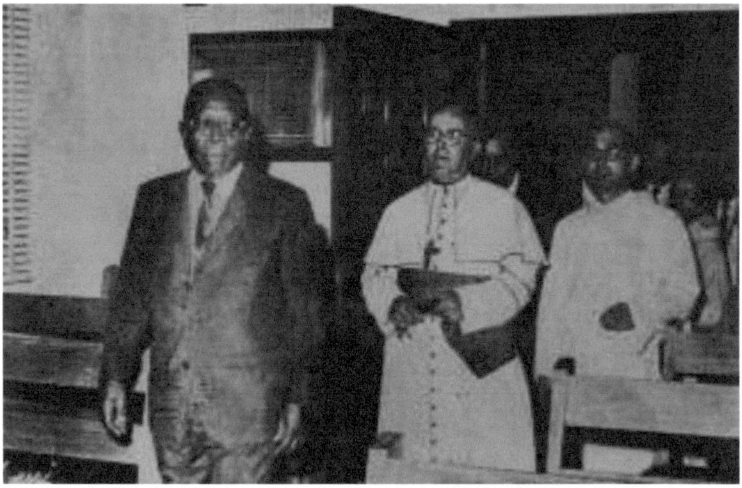

***President Tubman and Archbishop Francis Carroll at the dedication ceremony of the new institutions***

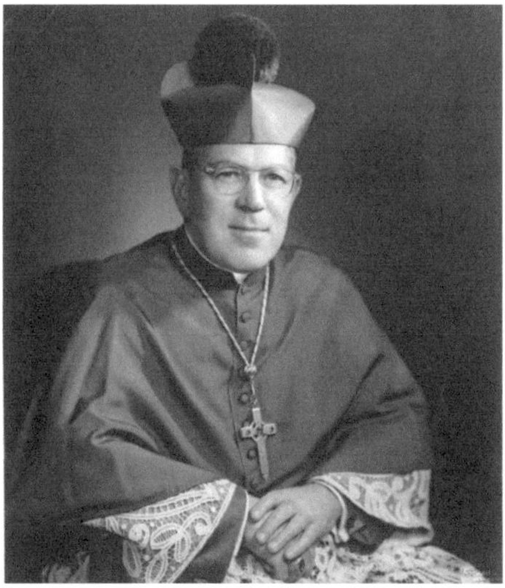

***Arch Bishop Francis D. Carroll***

By then, Bishop Francis D. Carroll was the apostolic nuncio to Liberia with the title of archbishop.

He was also the Ambassador of the Vatican in Liberia and therefore, helped to stear the entire construction of the two institutions, the hospital and the college.

In attendance at the formal groundbreaking ceremony were President Tubman, representing the government of Liberia, Archbishop Francis Carroll representing the Vatican, and the Italian Ambassador accredited near Monrovia- representing the Italian government.

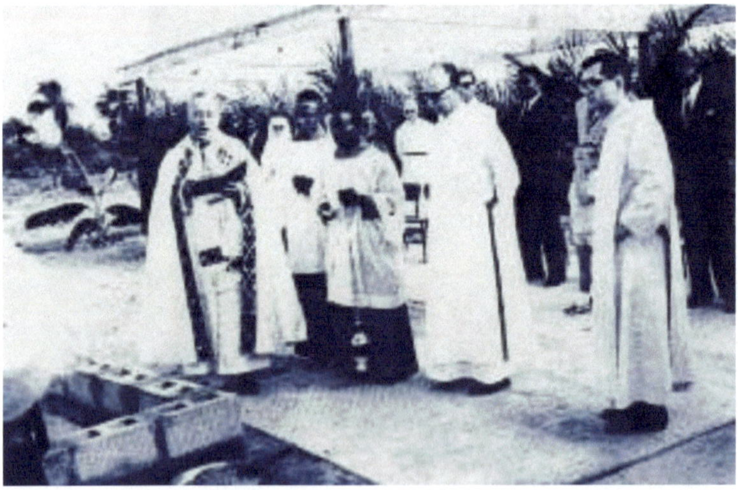

*Photo of the ground breaking ceremony*

# Chapter 5

## Turbulent (Ruffled) Beginnings

While the construction was in progress in 1966, the Dogliotti Foundation was all set to begin its task.

Therefore, in March of 1966, it commenced operations beginning with the Pre-medical School on the St. Patrick's High School campus, the present premises of the Stella Maris Polytechnic University (Don Bosco), located opposite the Ministry of Foreign Affairs on Capitol Hill.

**Professor Levi** was the first Italian Professor and Dean. All the original students were High School (secondary school) graduates and the lecturers were the St. Patrick's High School Holy Cross Brothers of the Catholic Diocese of Liberia.

## Objection to the Establishment of the Medical College

In every attempt to make a major change, the stakeholders do not always all agree on the details. The idea of a Liberian medical school was revolutionary. It would forever transform the health care landscape of the country.

There were key skeptic players that objected to the idea at its early stage, only because, in short sight and innocent faith, they thought the country was not ready for the venture. Foremost amongst that group were prominent Liberian medical doctors.

They doubted whether Liberia was ready to have a medical college, considering that, there was no existing infrastructure, nor the technical logistics, and manpower capacity to run the institution. They feared that at best, we might open a substandard training institution no better than an advanced nursing school.

Notwithstanding the doubts, President Tubman insisted the project go ahead. In furtherance thereof, after the construction was completed, a nationwide advertisement was made to recruit students.

The initial response was dismal probably because of confidence crisis. Very few Liberians were prepared to risk their future entering a Medical College in Liberia.

Apparently, even among the prospective student population, many doubted whether a medical college operating in Liberia would be equipped enough to train them.

During that era, going abroad- to the United States, other African countries, and Europe- for medical education was the brain-washed order of the day.

Of course, this doubt would in the future be dispelled by the advantages highlighted from the results of a WHO sponsored scientific study in 2006 at the University of Nairobi, Kenya.

The study compared the benefits of training doctors at home against training them abroad. The result revealed firstly that the financial costs associated with training doctors abroad and the loss of services (by failure to return) were way too high.

On the one hand, the disadvantages of studying abroad include;

1) *The cost of training is more expensive.*
2) *Many families will be separated.*
3) *The trainee's services are given to foreign countries and taxes are paid abroad, while in training.*
4) *There is a high probability of not returning home after study, or coming back only after retirement.*

This shows that the doctors' most productive years are being spent abroad, instead of at home, where it is most needed.

Conversely, the study showed that local trainings were more profitable and produced the following benefits as spelled out below:

1) *The training of doctors locally is cheaper*
2) *Locally trained doctors continue to give services while under training.*
3) *They mentor the lower-level students (paramedics and nurses) at low cost.*
4) *The chances are high for them to get married locally to their nationals.*
5) *If they eventually open their private practices upon graduating, they will provide employment for others, and continue to provide their uninterrupted services to their country.*
6) *They pay taxes at home, build, and stay to develop their country early*

Thus, the college recruited its first batch of students and started operations as a pre-medical school at St. Patrick's School Campus.

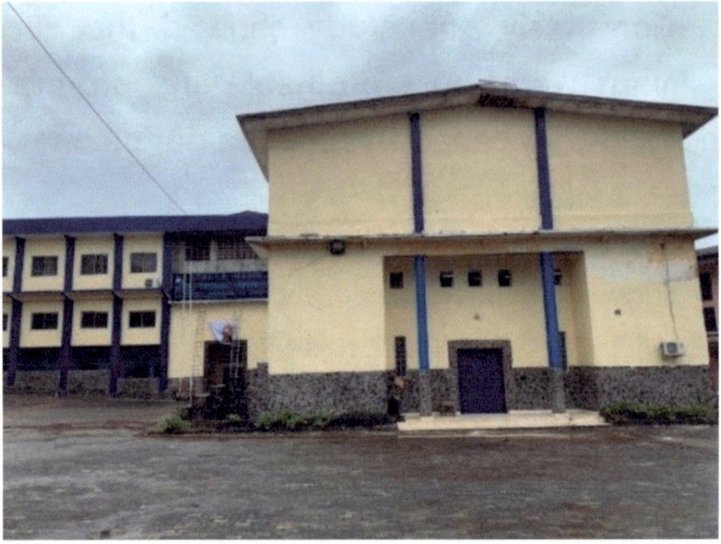

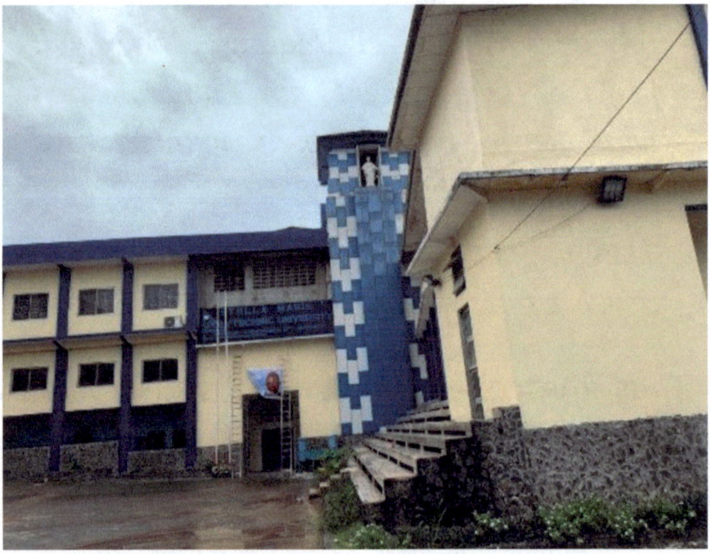

*Renovated Current campus 2022*

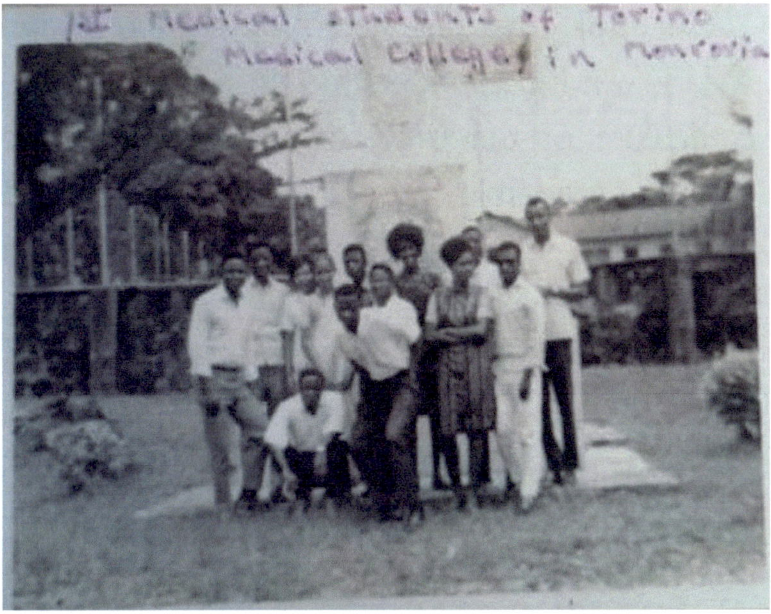

*Photo of the first pre medical students M-T-CM[3] taken in 1966 at the St. Patrick's High School Campus*

***Front**: (Sitting) Mensah-(**Bending**), Robert Kpoto – (**Back Standing L-R**) Gregory Okrokoto, Joseph Kabba, Julius Flowers, Sussama Kurien, Samuel Bowman, Maima Fahnbulleh-Freeman, Rose McCauley, Adolph Wagna, Richard Buxton, Engmann*

***Absent** were: Z. Sherman Adams and Benjamin Kajuah*

Majority of those that initially enrolled came from Maryland, Grand Cape Mount, Montserrado, and Lofa Counties. The foreign students admitted were mostly from Nigeria, Sierra Leone, and India.

---

[3] ***MTCM: Monrovia Torino College of Medicine**

In 1967, the pre-medical program of the college was incorporated into the science college curriculum of the University of Liberia as the seventh academic program and the second professional school (the Law School being the first).

Students therefore had to, transfer from the St. Patrick's School Campus to the next- door Capitol Hill campus of the University of Liberia.

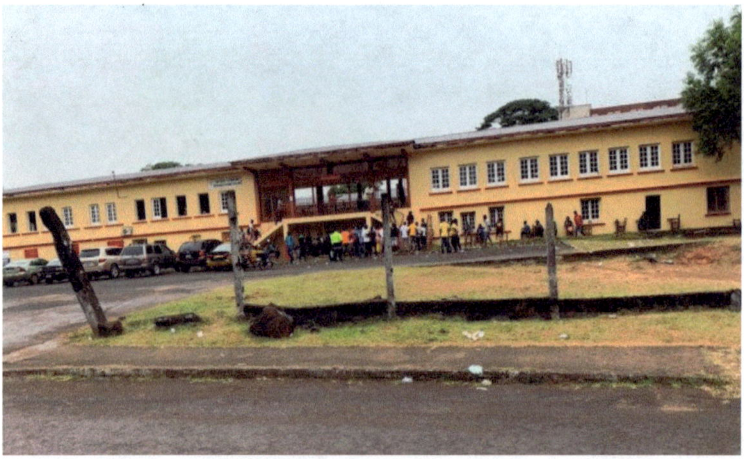

*University of Liberia Science College*

During the same year, the Monrovia- Torino Medical College and St. Joseph's Catholic Hospital edifices were formally completed, dedicated, and inaugurated.

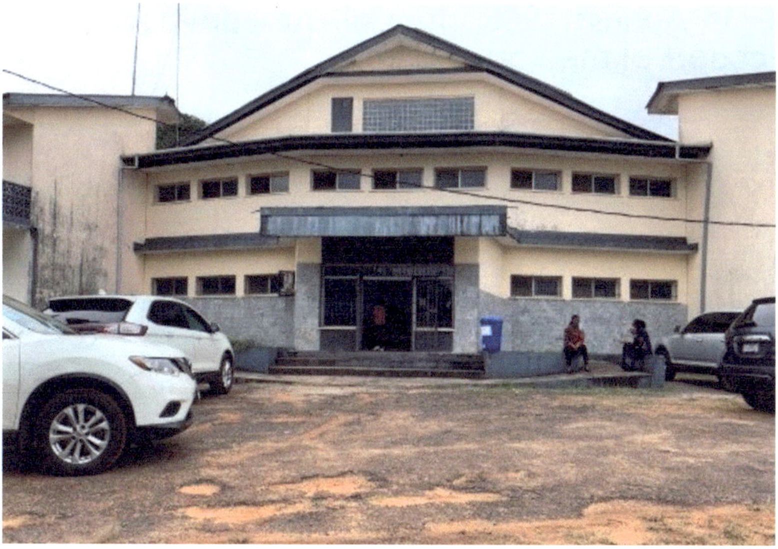

*The medical college building of AMD*

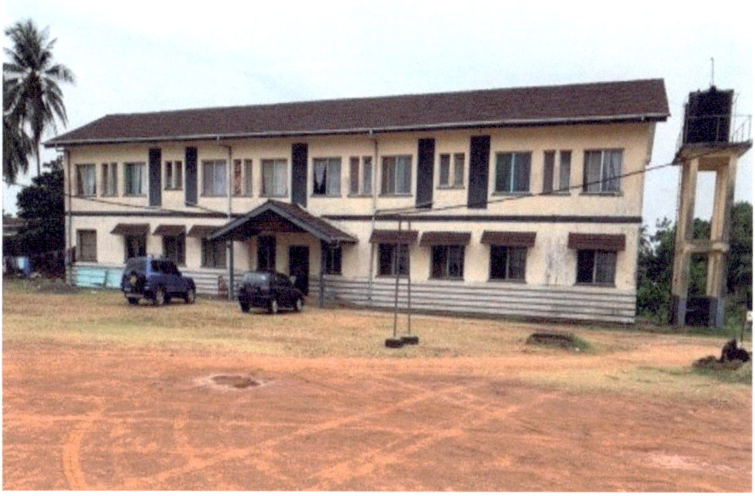

*Dormitory. The author's room was the first from the left, on the upper floor*

In August 1968, the College admitted its first cohort of medical students.

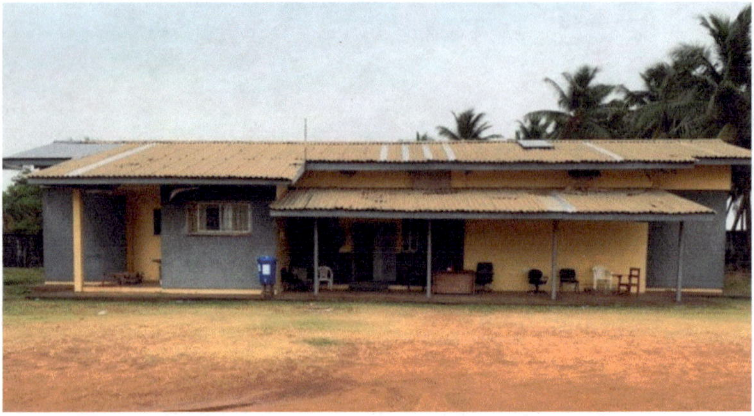

***Photo of the administrative building***

*The original home of the Italian administrator; now offices of the Dean and Staff*

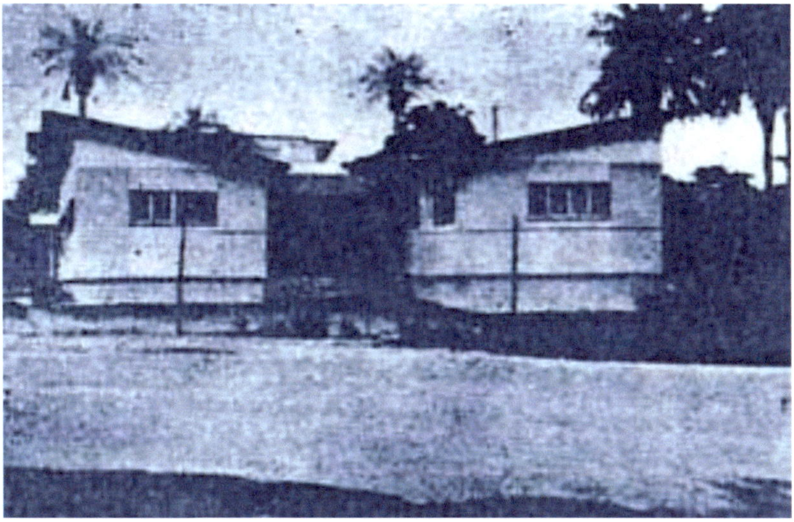

*The Original site of St. Joseph's Health Center near 24th Street, Tubman Blvd now, the Stryker Funeral Parlor*

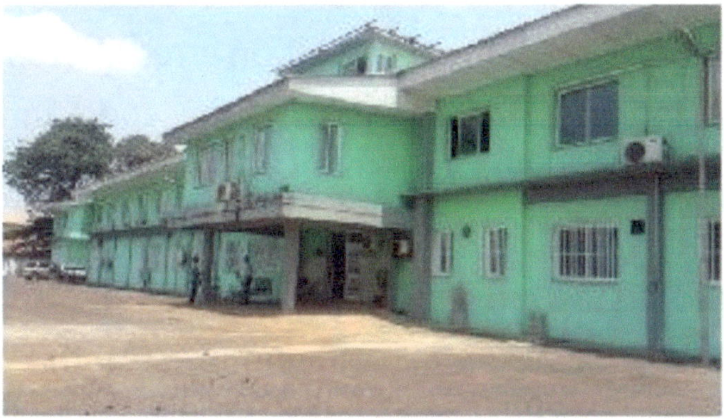

*Current St. Joseph's Catholic Hospital*

# Chapter 6

## Casting the Dices

The student population resembled a melting pot of nations with the spectrum of nationalities from across Liberia, Sierra Leone, Nigeria, and India. Against the backdrop of doubt in the country, the pioneer students who risked their future careers and entered the pre-medical school were: **Ziayue Sherman Adams, Samuel Bowman, Richard Boxton** (all from the St. Patrick's High School), and **Robert Momo Kpoto** (from the Laboratory High

School now William V.S. Tubman High). Others were **Kabbah** from Lofa; **Roseline Macaulay** and **Benjamin Kajuah** (Sierra Leone); **Susama Kurien** (India) but a resident of Harper, Maryland County); **Maima Fahnbuleh** (Cape Mount County); **Gregory Okrokoto** (Nigeria); **Julius Flowers** (Montserrado County), **Adolph Wagner, Mensah, and Timothy** (Harper, Maryland County).

***********

The first Administrator for the medical college was **Dr. Giuseppe Gautero** (Italian) from Torin. The first pre-medical lecturer and dean, **Professor Levi**, who eventually developed a kidney problem. We were told that he was born with only one kidney and therefore had to return home.

***********

At the end of the two-year pre-medical school, only six of the original fifteen students were successful to advance to the Medical College. They were:

1. *Z. Sherman Adams, Liberian*
2. *Samuel Bowman, Liberian*
3. *Richard Boxton, Liberian*
4. *Robert Momo Kpoto, Liberian*
5. *Susama Kurien, and Indian*
6. *Gregory Okrokoto, Nigerian*

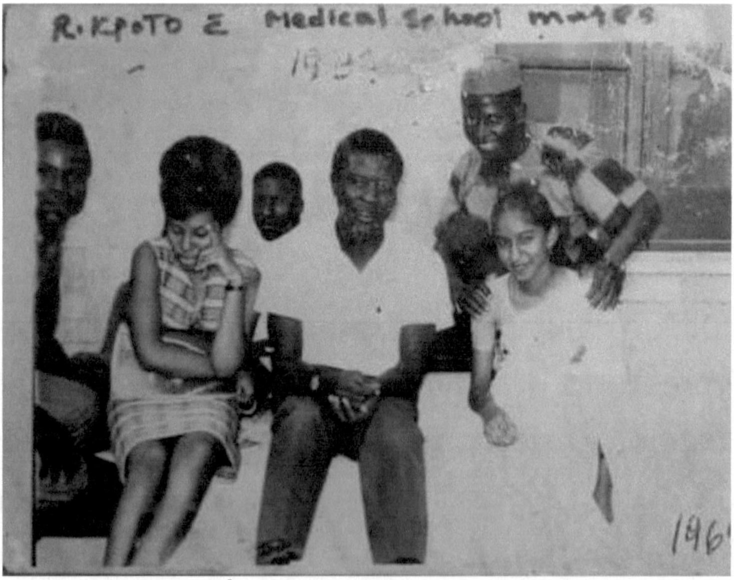


*(PHOTO of some 2nd year pre-med students) visiting the new college from the University of Liberia campus*
***L-R** Gregory Okrokoto, Julius Flowers, Richard Buxton, Benjamin Karjue, Sussama Kurien, Robert M. Kpoto- Back far right with cap and traditional attire*

The students who did not advance had either voluntarily left the university or transferred to other colleges. Some had even travelled outside the country before the term ended. We were so few first year cohorts that the administration delayed starting school and opted to advertise for additional students. The result was that, students from Cuttington College, joined us.

***********

This period coincided with the Nigerian-"Biafran" Civil War which ran from July 1967 to January 1970. Many young Nigerians fled their country, majority from the east and enrolled at the Cuttington College. Some of them constituted the additional recruits for the first cohort of the College in 1969. Joining us from Cuttington were: Emmanuel Kai-Lewis (Sierra Leone), Michael Ezundu, Dim Lazarus, Vincent Nwosa, Ambrose Okoye (all from eastern Nigeria) and Moses Seaton (from Lagos).

The total enrollment of the 1st cohort as of July 1969 was as follows:

*Moses Oluyemi Seton*
*Samuel G. Bowman*
*Michael Izundu*
*Emmanuel Sylvester Kai Lewis*
*Susama Kurien*
*Dim Lazarus*
*Vincent Isioma*
*Nwosa Ambros*
*Udozo Okoye*
*Gregory Oklokoto*
*Z. Sherman Adams*
*Robert M. Kpoto*
*Richard Buxton*

The first Dean succeeding Prof. Levi was **Prof. Gian Carlo Sethi**. He had difficulty speaking English and steering the affairs of the college.

At the end of 1969, the administrative situation of the college was chaotic, and in 1970, the University of Liberia took over control of the Medical College, completely.

The name of the College was changed from **Monrovia Torino College of Medicine** to **A.M. Dogliotti College of Medicine** in honor of Professor Achille Mario Dogliotti of the University of Torino, whose foundation was used to represent the Italian Government.

In 1971 when the John F. Kennedy Medical Center was inaugurated, it became the de facto teaching hospital (without any Legislative Act to so designate it) because the Catholic Hospital, which was originally built to serve as the teaching hospital, was now under the Catholic Diocese as their private missionary hospital. Almost all the faculties of the college were from Italy, majority from the University of Torino.

This sudden change of administrative structure from Italian to local staff was poorly planned (or not at all) and therefore very confusing. It later proved more challenging with unanticipated, stratified, administrative bottle-necks. The Italian Administration now nullified had no control over finances to operate. There was disarray in the college.

**The Impact that the University of Liberia take-over had on the First Cohort**

The confusion made the students of the first year so discouraged that majority except four of the original First Cohort decided to leave before the end of the academic year. The four students who remained were – Samuel Bowman, Michael Izundu, Moses Seaton, and Susana Korein.

Some of those that left returned home to Nigeria, others went to Europe, and all the Liberians, besides Bowman, left.

Sherman Adams got employed with (LAMCO) – Liberia-American Mining Company and Robert Kpoto returned to the regular undergraduate university program to complete his first college degree, because after the two-year Pre-med study, there was no academic certification earned.

The four students of the first cohort who continued in the program became the first to graduate in 1973. Amongst them was the only Liberian, *Dr. Samuel G. Bowman.* Others were *Dr. Michael Ezundu, Dr. Susama Korein*, and *Dr. Moses Seaton.*

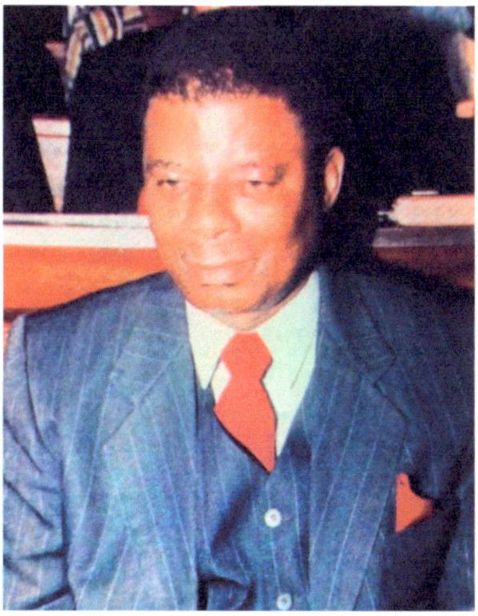

***Dr. Samuel Gbao Bowman***

At the end of the year in 1969 and before the academic year of 1970, the Liberian students who had left, Sherman Adams, Robert Kpoto and Richard Boxton- returned and decided to continue as the second cohort. They realized that staying away was not the best option for their dreams and ambitions to become medical doctors as they had not the financial resources needed to matriculate in another country.

By this time, additional students from Cuttington and other parts of Nigeria joined the college, constituting the 2nd cohort that went on to become the second graduates in 1974.

There were ten students in that class that graduated:

1. Ziayou Sherman Adams
2. Robert Momo Kpoto
3. Clemet Dafiluelo
4. Chuke Agu
5. Emmanuel Kai Lewis
6. Paul Menteh
7. Augustin Okonmah
8. Albert C. Okonkwo
9. Oyesola Afolabi Oyelayo
10. Ambrose Okoyeah

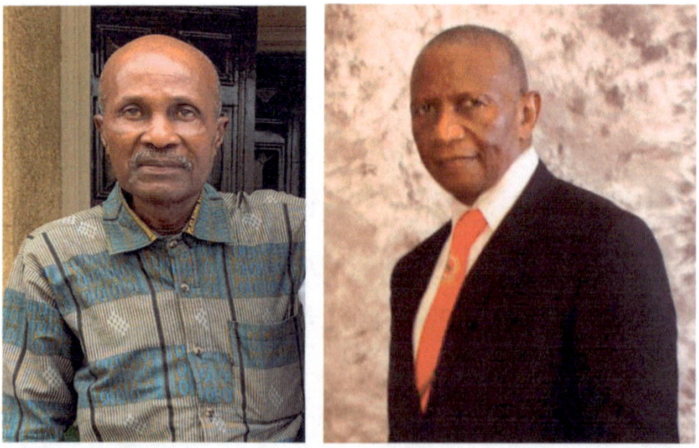

*Prof. Ziayou Sherman Adams and Prof. Robert Momo Kpoto, the only two Liberian pioneer students alive. They (graduated with the second cohort).*

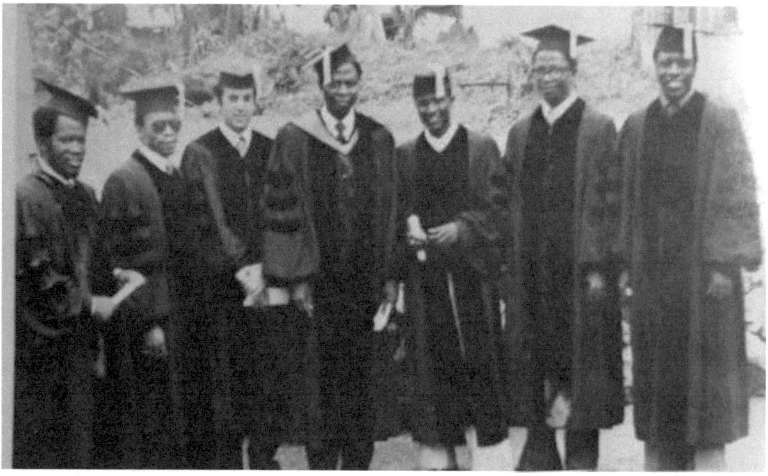

*Prof. Daramola and some members of the graduating class of the second cohort – 1974*
***L-R**; Emmanuel Kai Lewis, Clement Dafiluelo, an Italian faculty member, Dean Daramola, Z. Sherman Adams, Robert M. Kpoto, and Albert Okonkwo*

After graduation and internship, a Two (2) year national service was mandatory for all students on government sponsored scholarships.

Dr. Kpoto was assigned in Zorzor, (Curran Lutheran Hospital) in Lofa County while the others were assigned to different regions of the country.

*************

Following the graduation of the second class the college had a stream of graduates (see

Appendix 2) despite the administrative and logistic challenges that bedeviled the institution. Concomitantly there was a very fast-turnover of deans as the transition from the Italians to Liberians accelerated. (See appendix 5 for deans of medical college)

There were few short-lived Liberian deans and interim deans that took over from the Italians. The first Liberian Dean of the College was Dr. Edwin Murray Barclay, (January 1971) a former Minister of Health.

Dean Barclay's administration was turbulent, rugged, and stagnant. He was replaced by Prof. Teawor Daramola, a Nigerian professor married to a Liberian - Florence McClain Daramola. Mrs. Daramola was a Professor of Physiology and the niece of Liberia's 19th President, William Tolbert.

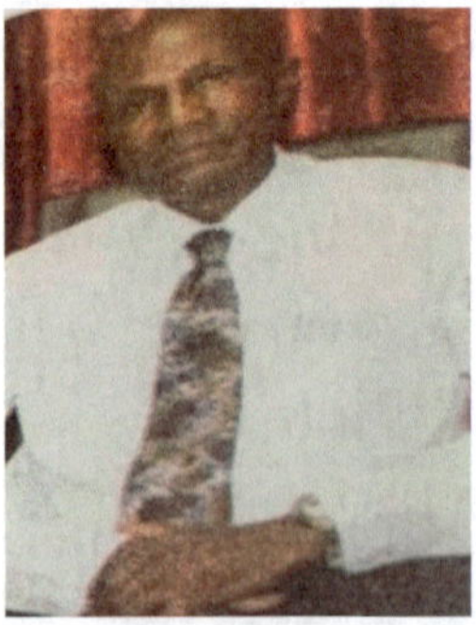

***Dean Edwin Murray Barclay***

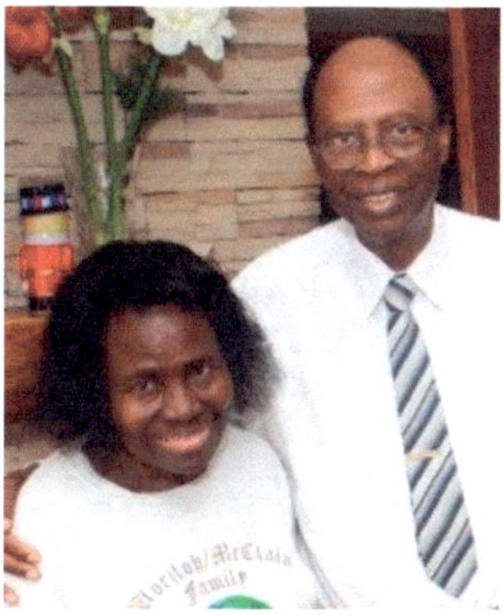

***Dean Teawor Daramola & Prof. Florence McClain Daramola***

Thus, with Prof. Daramola's recruitment as Dean of the College, we fortunately gained two professors at once.

Professor Daramola was very efficient, dynamic, and proactive. When he took over the college, majority of the students were foreigners.

He disagreed with the policy that students were placed on the Liberian government scholarships regardless of their nationalities. So, he set out to transform the situation by introducing the quota system in which only 30% of space was allotted to non-Liberians.

It was from this policy that the College progressively recruited more Liberians.

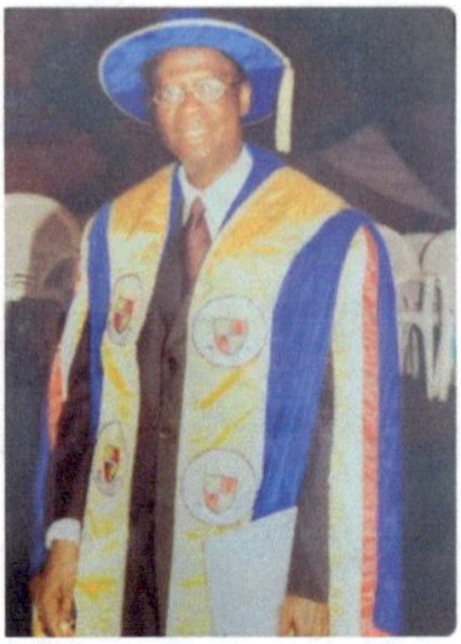

***Professor Teawor Daramola (as Provost of the University of Ilorin after her returned to Nigeria)***

As observed earlier, the first and second cohorts had only one and two Liberian graduates respectively. But as a result of Professor Daramola's restructuring of the system, there was gradual arithmetic progression in the number of Liberian students admitted in the college.

**Now over 90%** of enrollments in the institution are Liberians. Beginning with the first four graduates in 1973, the A.M. Dogliotti College of Medicine has trained **602** doctors up to the publication of this book. (See Appendix 2)

They are deployed all through the length and breadth of the country, giving health care services in our hospitals, and simultaneously training other doctors and paramedical professionals.

> *It is my hope that the A.M. Dogliotti College of Medicine will in the future also export doctors to other countries.*

**Dean Festus Moley Halay** succeeded Dean Daramola in 1977. He was a Liberian surgeon. Dean Halay was trained at Howard University in Washington D.C. He hails from Lofa County.

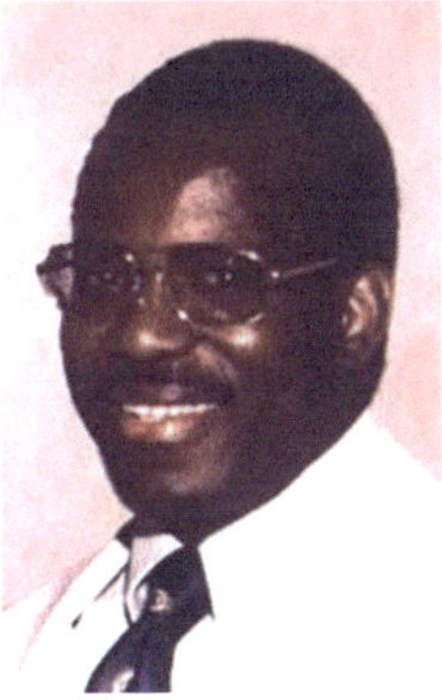

***Dean Festus Moley Halay***

Dean Halay was one of the hardest working and student-welfare-oriented deans. He left in 1983 for family reasons and was succeeded by Dr. **Wilmot Dennis**, the first Liberian physiotherapist.

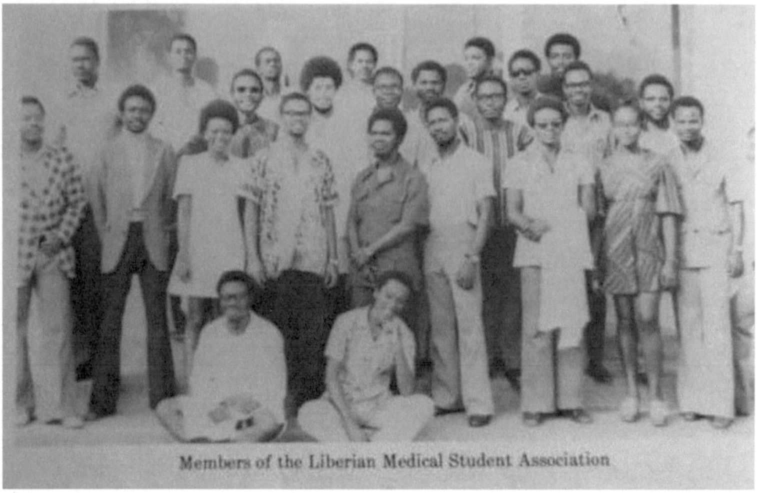


***Some members of the Liberian Medical Students Association***

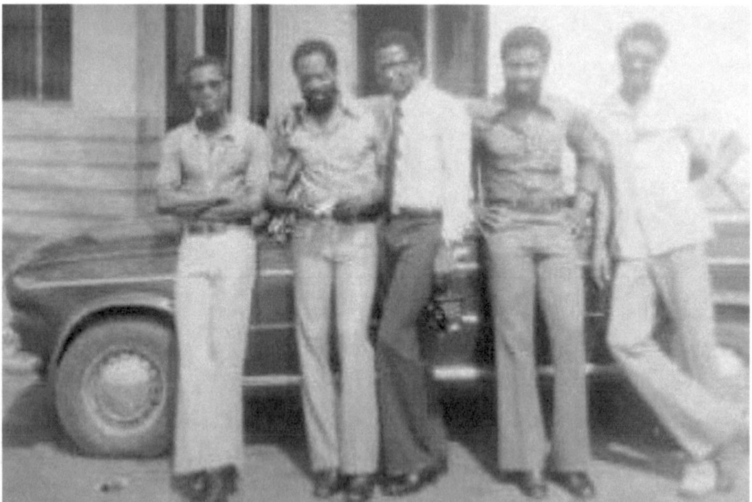

***The author with some friends; L-R: Z. Sherman Adams, Antonio Viddy (Angola), Robert Kpoto, Oyesola A. Oyelaya (Nigeria), Okpawoye Adebayo (Nigeria), taken in front of the medical college resident building.***

# Section Two

## THE CIVIL WAR AND ITS IMPACT ON MEDICAL EDUCATION

# Chapter 7

## The Impact of the Civil Crisis on Medical Education

The civil crisis, which exploded in December of 1989 damaged the nation. I say exploded because the crisis was in the making several years before and only needed a catalyst to ignite it.

The death toll rose to the tune of nearly a quarter of a million, over the 14 years of its three-phased episodes. These spasmodic episodes of the crisis interrupted the training of medical doctors for ten cumulative years divided metaphorically into:

World War I (1989 to 1995)
World War II (1998 to 2000)
World War III (2003 to 2004)

During these periods, graduations for medical doctors were interrupted. As a result of these delays, some doctors, including civil servants, and officials of government advocated for the official closure of the College, because the war depleted our capacity for quality training.

But thanks to the resistance and resilience of noble colleagues like **Prof. Benson Barh,** who was then acting Dean of the college, and the late **Prof. Arthur Lewis**, Chairman of the Faculty of Pharmacy, the college was not closed. These two strong professors of the College deserve commendation for refusing to officially close the institution. Prof. Robert M. Kpoto joined the chorus of non-closure and supported the resistance group.

They feared that once the college was officially closed, it would be more difficult to reopen. They believed it was better to have it even intermittently operating, until there was help for rehabilitation and improvement. This decision proved right in the end.

The reason of their rejection to the closure is reminiscent of the reason of Elijah Johnson's rejection to accept help from the British. We read in our Liberian History about one of the early battles between the Settlers and the tribal people.

It is written that, as the war raged and it appeared that the tribal people were winning, the British arrived with an offer to help the Settlers fight. This was a most attractive and welcomed bait; except that in return, the British wanted to put up their flag, meaning, they'd have territorial claim.

At that point, one great Settler (Eli Johnson) said ***"We want no flagstaff put up here. It will cost us more to take down than it will to whip the natives".*** That critical statement and decision helped to save the independence of Liberia.

**********

The 1989 civil war resulted into infrastructural damage, pillage, and destruction to the entire fabric of the institution. The greatest loss indeed was that of the hemorrhage of professional manpower. Most of the specialists and faculty members fled for their lives; thereby creating a technical anemia. The college practically went into shock, and intermittently into coma.

Then suddenly came a savior after the first episode of the crisis- (World War I), when the **Arch Bishop Michael Frances** made cash donations, on behalf of the Catholic Church of Liberia, to rehabilitate the College.

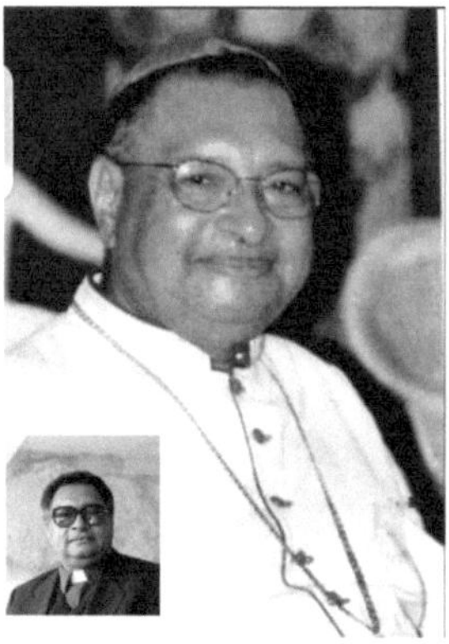

***Arch Bishop Michael Frances***

Additional support from World Health Organization helped to refurbish most of the damaged buildings, thus reviving hope and infusing new life in the college.

The infrastructural dilapidation was just one of the many problems. The college was still plagued with other issues, namely, the lack of operational logistics, qualified work force, security, and of course, good administration.

During those difficult years, I continued to give scholarships (which included the payment of their school fees and monthly stipends) to needy students in the Colleges of Pharmacy and Medicine. The students qualified based on their dire needs, not academic excellence. Many students took advantage of the scholarships.

Fundamentally, for me, it was the realization that most of the efforts made to support the college would have been in vain if the students were too hungry to study or too busy looking for food to eat and missed classes. Those indeed were some of our post war realities.

Over the years, as the country gradually experienced peace, the college became stronger in infrastructure, logistics, and manpower capacity; especially as locally trained doctors, including those from abroad, started returning to help along with the international community.

Prominent among the Liberian doctors who returned home from the diaspora and made immense contribution to the rehabilitation and development of the medical college was Professor Vuyu Kanda Golakai, a general surgeon, an academician, and former Chief Executive Officer of the JFK Medical Center.

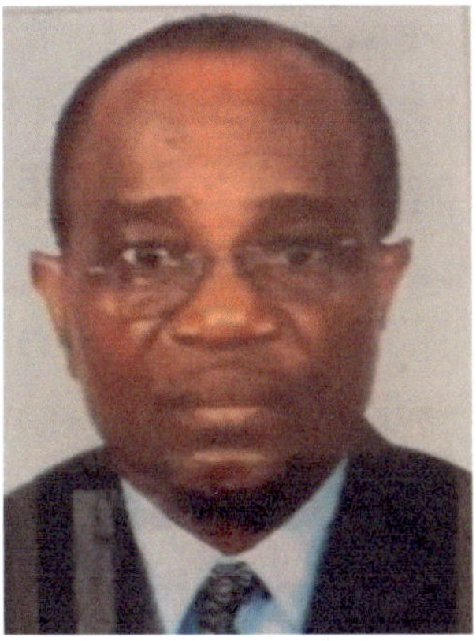

***Prof. Vuyu Kanda Golakai***
*General Surgeon*

His arrival was very timely, as he had a wealth of professional and administrative experience. He therefore enjoyed the blessing and good will of his friend and former classmate, Dr. Emmet Dennis, who was now President of the University of Liberia.

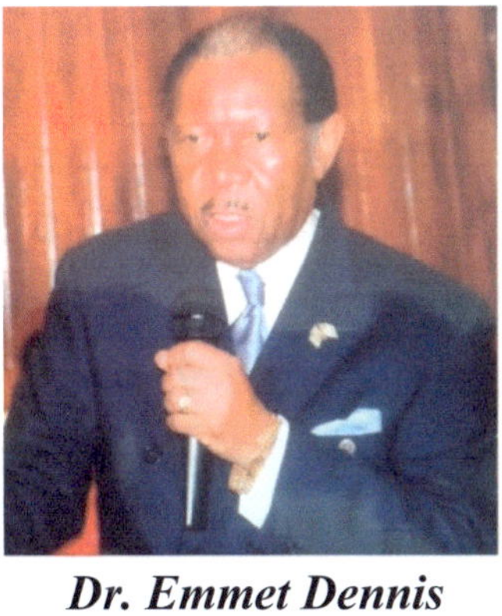

***Dr. Emmet Dennis***
*President of the Universit of Liberia*

Dr. Dennis appointed him Dean of the Medical College and for the first time to a second new position of Vice President for Health Sciences.

Armed with these portfolios, Professor Golakai, along with a team sent by the Italian Government, revised the curriculum of the college, rehabilitated the anatomy lab, the library, student dormitory and completed the staff quarters for visiting professors.

He set up the computer lab and initiated an online portal allowing students, for the first time, to follow lectures outside of the classrooms. He advocated for and obtained an increase in the allowance of the medical students.

By the time of his retirement, the emeritus professor had doubled the post- war college student enrollment and the number of full-time professors among his many achievements.

There was now a gradual, visible improvement in the general post-war healthcare, measured by a reduction in the patient/doctor ratio and the decline in the infant morbidity and mortality rates. This was because there were now more trained doctors who took over medical facilities across the country.

Despite these local gains, the post war slump in the economy made it difficult for graduating doctors to go abroad for needed specialist training, a sector critically demanded by necessity.

It was then that the long-incubated conversation to start training our own specialists was hatched and became more relevant in all the social strata of the country, from the grassroots, the technocrats, to the politicians. Therefore, fertilizing the soil for the planting of our own post graduate medical college.

# Section Three

## THE LIBERIA POSTGRADUATE COLLEGE OF PHYSICIANS ANS SURGEONS

# Chapter 8

## College of Peers

At the end of the 1989 civil war that lasted over 14 years, the economy got worse, making Liberia almost a failed state, and therefore the cost of sending doctors abroad for post graduate specialization, almost prohibitive.

The average Liberian patient couldn't afford the cost of going out of the country for specialized medical treatments, as there were very few specialist doctors in the country.

This precarious situation accentuated the serious consideration for the establishment of a Post Graduate College of Medicine in the country; one that would train specialists for the counties and greatly improve the national healthcare system, train trainers, and boost the economy.

The dire need and practicality of Liberia having the ability to train its own specialists, culminated into the birth of the Liberia Post Graduate College of Physicians and Surgeons (LCPS).

The history of LCPS has similarities to that of the West African College of Surgeons (WACS), in that the groundbreaking ideas to start both institutions, though more than half a century apart and completely independent of each other, were hatched by young graduates from foreign medical institutions.

In the case of WACS, in the 1960s, a young Cameroonian, Dr. Victor Anomah Ngu, after completing fellowship training in surgery in Britain, decided to return home. While in the ship on his way back home, he met and discussed the need for a forum for surgeons in practice in West Africa with a retired British surgeon Charles Bowesman who was also returning to Ghana. Dr. Ngu believed that a West African College of medical professionals was important and needed for the sub-region.

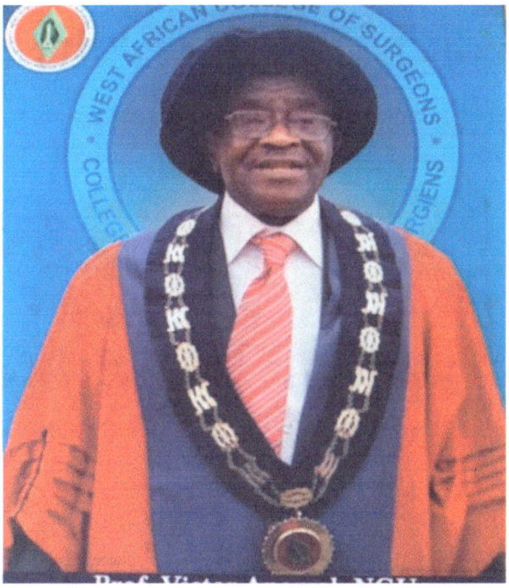


***Dr. Victor Anomah Ngu***

He went to Nigeria and shared the idea with his professors who bought and developed it into what is now the single largest body of medical professionals in the West African sub-region- The West African College of Surgeons (WACS).

Similarly, the idea to start a Post Graduate Medical College in Liberia was catalyzed by a young Liberian, Dr. Abraham Saah Borbor.

Dr. Borbor completed his Post Graduate Medical Training in Internal Medicine in Tanzania, East Africa.

He returned home in September 2006 and was appointed Head of the Department of Internal Medicine at the John F. Kennedy (JFK)Medical Center.

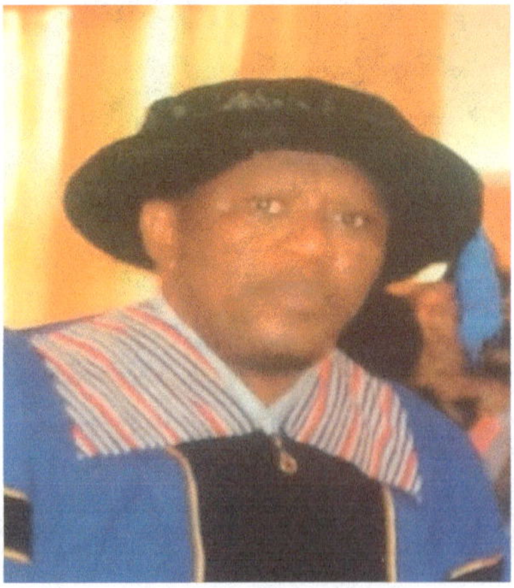

***Dr. Abraham Saah Borbor***

At the time, I was Acting Chief Medical Officer (CMO) of JFK and a professor of Orthopedic Surgery in the Department of Surgery. It was during one of my departmental rounds that the young Dr. Borbor proposed that Liberia should establish its own Post Graduate Medical Training Program.

An idea that until then, of course, had been ruminating in the minds of some healthcare policymakers including me. I had had similar conversations in the past with Dr. Ivan B. Camanor, who was the Chief Medical Officer and Deputy Minister of Health in 1986.

Dr. Borbor advanced his idea by telling me, "Chief", in his usual humble way of addressing his seniors, "I can bring the curriculum from Dar es-Salaam, Tanzania, where I studied".

***The idea*** seemed great, so I agreed. He, immediately translated his words into action.

His idea, like that of Dr. Ngu of WACS, could not have come at a better time when post-war Liberia critically needed medical specialists.

Immediately, the proposal was accepted and I scheduled the first meeting that was held at the J.F.K. Medical Center Administration Office of Dr. **James Tomaken**, who was the country representative Staff of the Clinton Foundation.

Present at that first meeting in 2009 were Dr. Abraham Borbor, Prof. Joseph R. Njoh from Nigeria (whom I had recently recruited in the Department of Internal Medicine at the Medical Center), and me- Acting CMO.

Also, in attendance were both the immediate past and current deans of the A.M. Dogliotti College of Medicine - Dr. Benson Barh and Dr. Tarbeh Freeman, Sr. respectively.

A subsequent meeting was called at which time Dr. Emmet Dennis, President of the University of Liberia was invited for his advice on whether the new college should be under the University board or autonomous. Dr. Dennis clarified that under the University, the postgraduate certification would be a Masters degree and that the administration would be subject to the University Administration.

On the other hand, if a clinical postgraduate certificate (diplomate membership or fellowship) like those of the sub-regional West African colleges is the goal then, an autonomous college should be the option. Following these clarifications and advice, the committee unanimously decided to have the college autonomous and therefore wrote a proposal to Dr. Gwengali, Minister of Health for his consideration and advice.

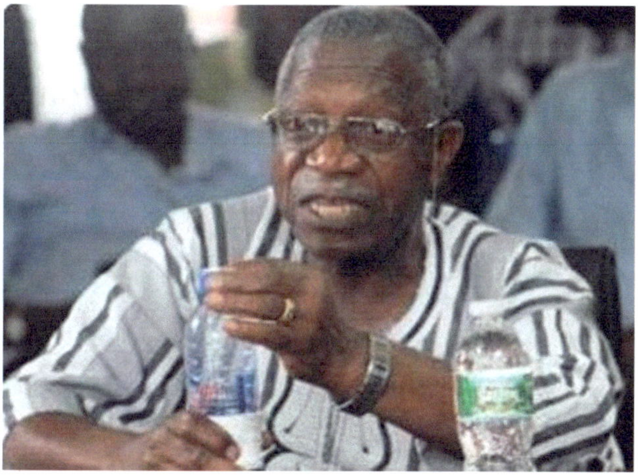

*Dr. Walter Gwenigale, Minister of Health, RL*

Dr. Gwenigale, at that crucial, immediate, post war period, was was actively sourcing ways to get Specialists into the country hospitals. He immediately formed two committees.

1. The Technical Working Committee headed by Dr. Bernice Dahn Chief Medical Officer/Deputy Minister of Health

2. The Advisory Committee comprising - Prof. Robert M. Kpoto (Chair), Prof. Vuyu Kanda Golakai, Dr. Benson Barh, and Dr. Walter Gwenigale exofficio

The technical working group headed by Dr. Dahn along with some other Committee members subsequently visited Ghana and Nigeria in the sub- region to study the West Africa Model of local Post Graduate Medical Training.

This was followed up with reciprocal visits by representatives from West African College of Surgeons (WACS) and the West African College of Physicians (WACP) comprising the Secretary General of WACS, Prof. Clement Wanwolo (Nigeria), along with Prof. Dr/Dr. Broby from Kwami Nkrumah University of Science and Technology (KNUST) (Ghana), Prof. Gladys Amposah, (Anesthesiologist), (Ghana), and the, Secretary General of WACP Prof. Bernard Nkum (Ghana) and others.

The Liberian delegation included:

1. Dr. Bernice Dahn
2. Prof. Robert M. Kpoto
3. Prof. Vuyu Golakai
4. Dr. Stephen Kennedy
5. Dr. Roseda Marshall
6. Dr. Benjamin Harris
7. Dr. Moses Massaquoi
8. Dr. John Mulbah
9. Dr. Billy Johnson
10. Dr. Nyankoi Kargbo

The team along with senior departmental heads and policy makers, had a three-day working retreat from August 23rd to 25th 2012 at Wulki Farm in Careysburg, Margibi County.

They brainstormed and carved out the template that would eventually guide the infant college in its Training Program. They designated seven training hospitlas across the country:

**Montserrado County**

JFK Medical Center

Redemption Hospital

ELWA Hospital

**Bong County**

Phebe Hospital/C. B. Dunbar Hospital

**Nimba County**

Jackson F. Doe Memorial Hospital

**Lofa County**

Tellwoyan Hospital

**Margibi County**

Du Side Hospital, Firestone

**Maryland County**

J. J. Dossen Hospital

The committees worked tirelessly, along with the LMDA, and submitted a bill to the legislature for an Act that was passed into law establishing the Liberia Postgraduate College of Physicians and Surgeons (LCPS) in December 2012 and signed by President Ellen Johnson Sirleaf in May of 2013.

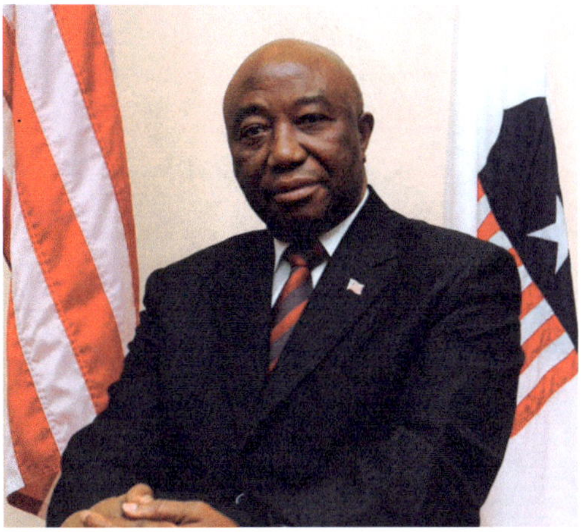

***Vice President Joseph Nyumah Boakai***

Subsequently, on September 30, 2013, His Excellency Ambassador Joseph Nyumah Boakai successfully launched the Liberia Postgraduate College of Physicians and Surgeons (LCPS) at the Ministry of Health Conference Room. The first interim executive officers of the college were:

***Dr. Roseda E. Marshall - President (Physician)***

***Prof. Robert M. Kpoto – 1st VP (Surgeon)***

***Dr. Benjamin Harris– 2nd VP (Physician)***

***Dr. Stephen B. Kennedy- Secretary General (Physician)***

***Dr. Rose Macauley – Honorary Treasurer (Physician)***

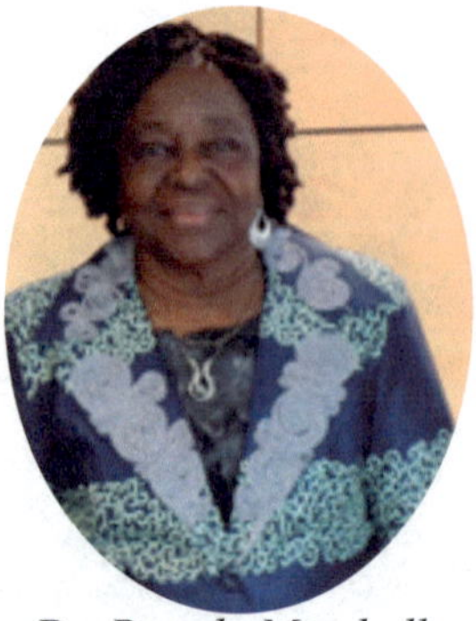

*Dr. Roseda Marshall*
*President*

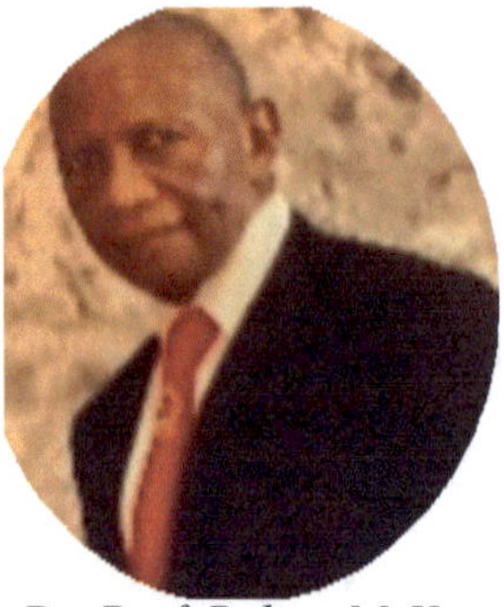

*Dr. Prof. Robert M. Kpoto*
*1st VP (Surgery)*

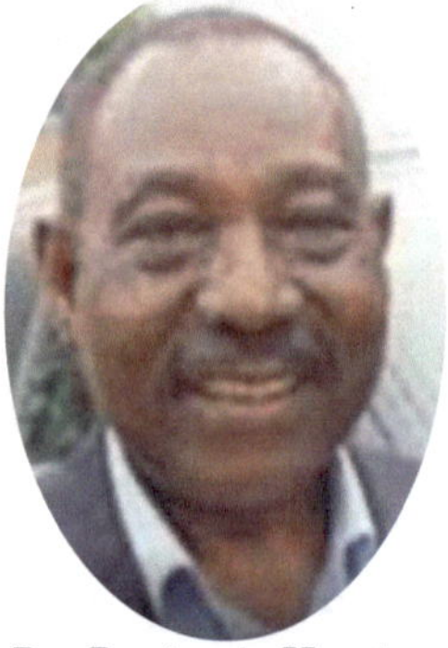

*Dr. Benjamin Harris*
*2nd VP (Physician)*

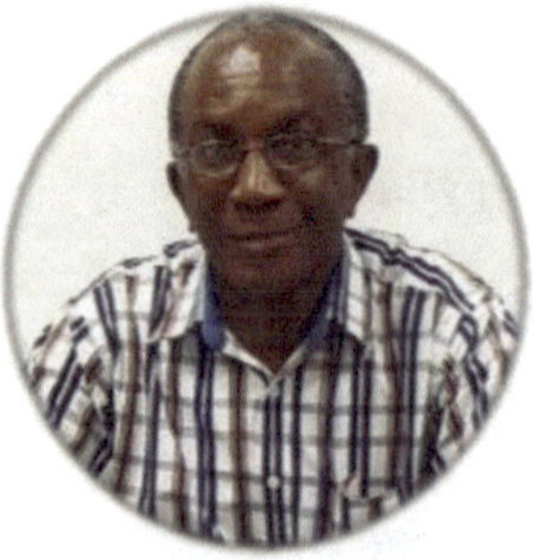

*Dr. Steve Kennedy*
*Secretary General*

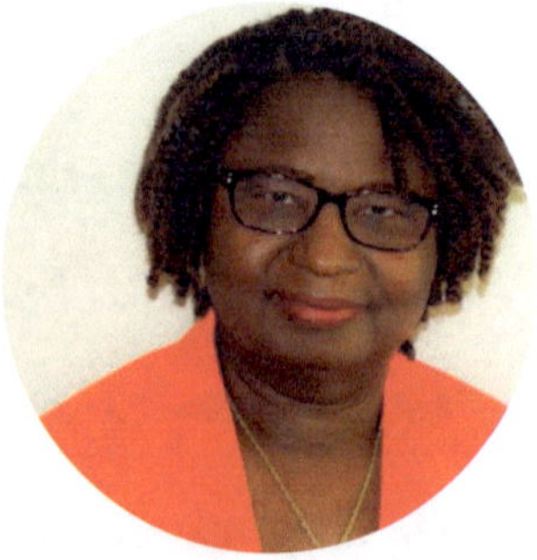

*Dr. Rose Macauley*
*Honorary Treasurer*

*********

On March 15, 2014, His Honor Vice President Joseph N. Boakai inducted the five executive officers along with the initial 55 foundation fellows admitted by the college. They came from the four faculties, Surgery, Obstetrics/Gynecology, Medicine, and Pediatrics (see Appendix 9)

This was followed by the recruitment of the first cohort of 19 residents distributed almost equally among the initial four faculties:

| No. | Faculty | Chair |
|---|---|---|
| 1. | Surgery (5 residents) | (Dr. Lawrence Sherman) Prof. Vaani Freeman[5]** |
| 2. | Obstetrics & Gynecology (5 residents) | Dr. John Mulbah |
| 3. | Internal Medicine (5 residents) | (Dr. Abraham Borbor) Prof. Joseph Njoh[6]*** |
| 4. | Pediatrics (4 residents) | Dr. Sia Camanor |

[5] Was replaced upon (unfinished tenure)

[6] Was replaced due to death.

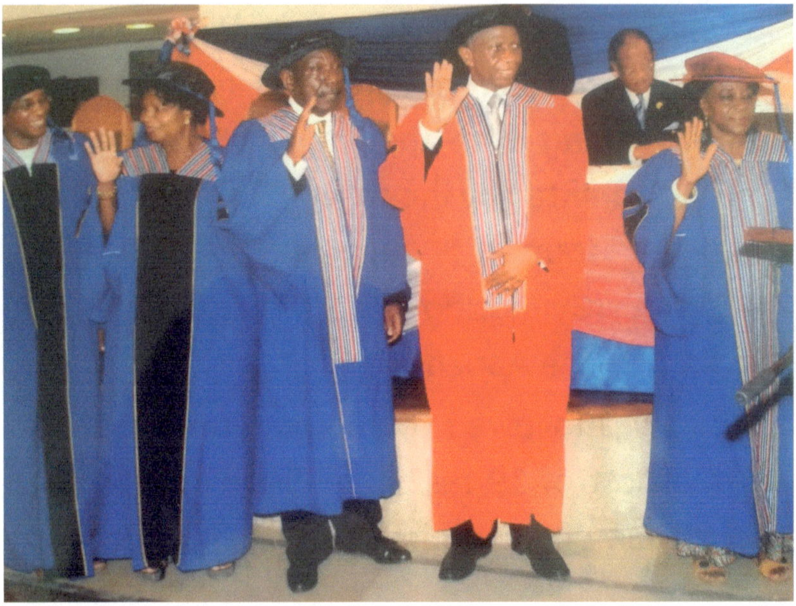

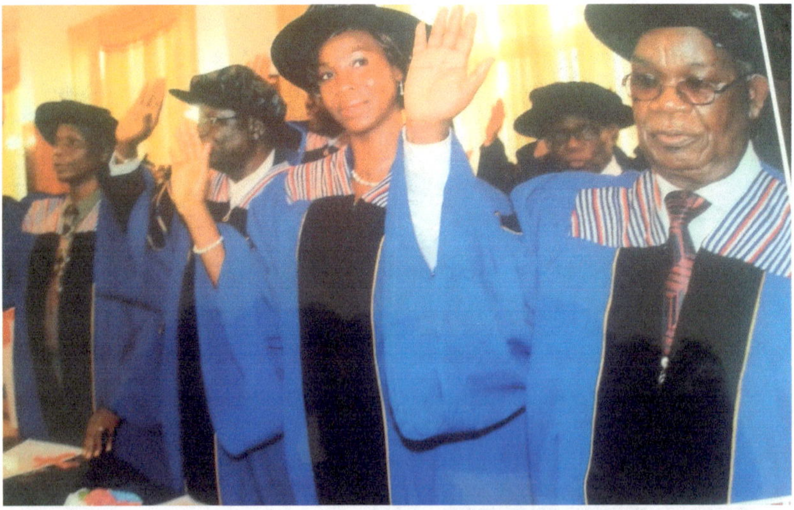

*Induction ceremony of the Executives and Foundation Fellows by His Excellency Ambassador Joseph Nyuman Boakai, Vice President, Republic of Liberia.*

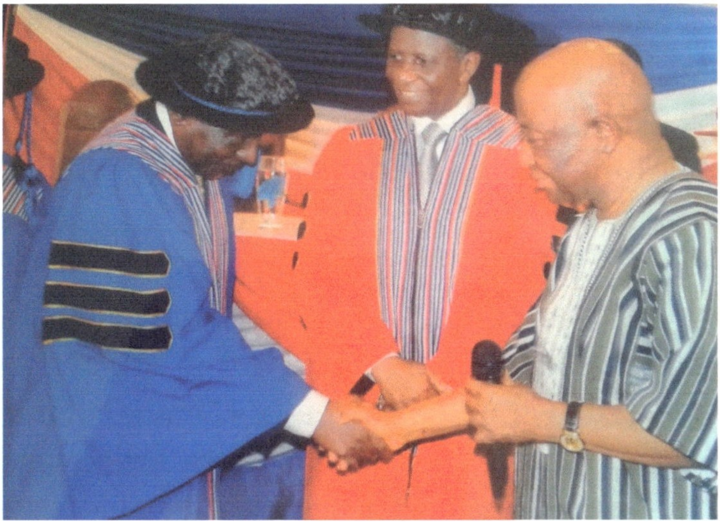

To immortalize Dr. Borbor's legacy for the ground breaking contribution to specialist postgraduate medical training and improving national health care delivery, the Liberia College of Physicians and Surgeons have set out an annual lecture series called ***Dr. Abraham Saah Borbor Lecture.*** It runs in his honor at every convocation of the college.

The beginning for the new college was not without challenges. Resources (material, human, and financial) were limited. Before the college could get any budgetary funding from the government, it had to struggle on its own. Fortunately, upon a request of the CMO, Dr. Bernice Dahn, Dr. Gwenigale the Minister approved funds for the support of the initial college operations. Not long after, the legislature gave budgetary allocation and then the World Bank provided additional support.

At the onset, Liberians chaired and staffed all the four faculties. The college designed a three-year Specialist Training Program for all the four disciplines. At the end of the first three years, the first cohort of doctors graduated as specialists with the Degree of Membership in Surgery, Internal Medicine, Obstetrics and Gynecology, and Pediatrics.

Since its launching in 2013, the College has had **six (6) cohorts of graduating specialists** in their respective disciplines. To date (2022) **One Hundred Ten (110)** specialists have been trained.

Moreover, in designing the college program, a mechanism is in place for the creation of additional faculties, as and when needed.

With special financial support from the World Bank, American universities partners and NGO's, the college has added, all together three additional faculties, summing up to seven (7).

| The 3 New Faculties | **Ophthalmology** | **Psychiatry** | **Family Medicine** |
|---|---|---|---|
| **Chair** | Dr. Niranja Pehere | Dr. Babawale Ojediran | Dr. David Okiror |
| **Sponsor** | ***LV –Prasad Eye Institute India*** Supported by Lion Club International | Boston University Medical Center-USA | USAID –SIM and other collaborating parties |
| **Lead Establisher** | ***Prof. Gullapalli Nageswara*** RAO Ophthalmologis t Founder & CEO | Prof. David H. Henderson Psychiatrist | Dr. Richard A. Sacra Family Medicine (MISSIONARY EBOLA SURVIVOR) |
| **Photo** | 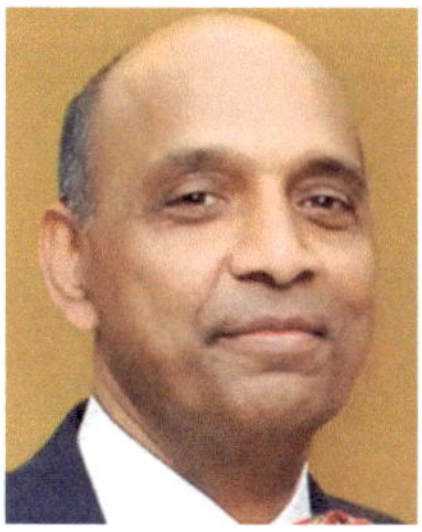 | 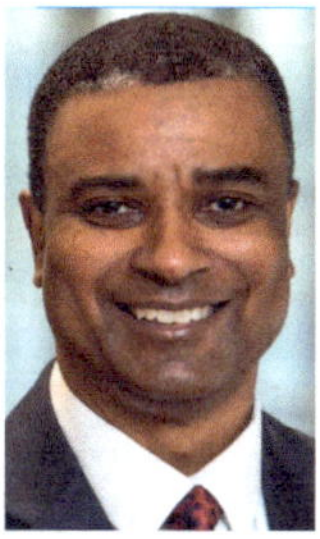 | 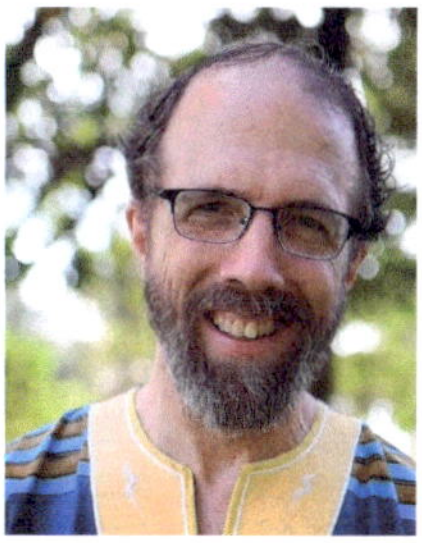 |

The College during the presidency of Professor Robert M. Kpoto received Special Financial Aid from the Government of Liberia in 2017 and sent **seventeen** (17) residents out of the country to specialize in disciplines that were not specifically offered at LCPS.

These included Orthopedic Surgery, Urology, Otorhinolaryngology (ENT), Pediatric Surgery Anesthesiology, Pathology, Emergency Medicine and Psychiatry (afterwards, this Faculty was added) to the college.

Currently, the college has embarked on a Fellowship Training Program and concomitantly pursuing the West Africa College of Surgeons and Physicians for reciprocity and harmonization ofthe curricula in the training of Specialists that would practice anywhere in the Sub-region.

In furtherance of that harmonization agenda, supported by West Africa Health Organization (WAHO) a QUINTAPATITE group of colleges with common goals for harmonization of medical education and services in the subregion has been formed and presently comprises:

1. Liberia local college
2. Ghana local college
3. Nigeria local college
4. WACS
5. WACP

One of the major goals of the LCPS now is to establish its own fellowship program and have sub-regional reciprocal college accreditation and recognition of training facilities (teaching hospitals) and trainees by both WACS and WACP for Specialist Training.

Meanwhile, the performance of our Residents in sub-regional Specialist Exams has been outstanding and commendable.

Our college will continue with its own local fellowship training trajectory as it persues and awaits the consummation of the subregional reciprocity from WACS and WACP.

**Photo after the 1st membership exit exam – surgery**
**Venue: ELWA Hospital**

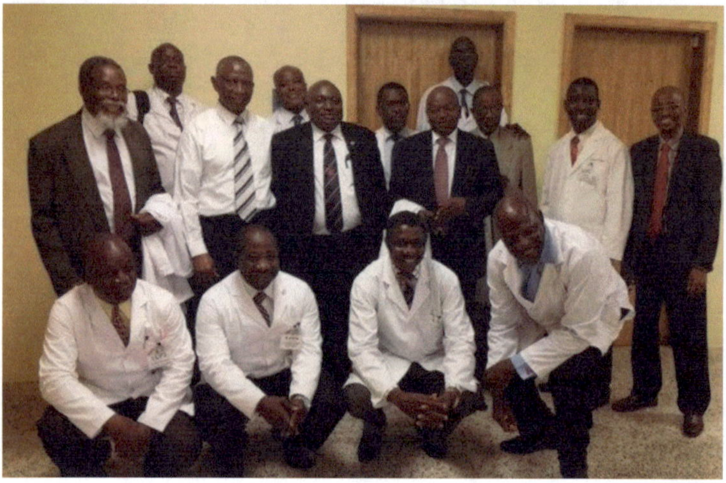

***Sitting*** *(L-R) Graduating Class: Dr. Saygbeh Vanyanbah, Dr. Suleimanu Konneh, Dr. Terseer Utam, and Dr. J. Fallah Moses*

***Standing Examination Faculty****: (L-R)* ***Front****: Prof. Nkruma Mills; Prof. Robert M. Kpoto; Prof. King David T. Yaweh; Prof. Varnee Freeman; Dr. Jerry Brown; Dr. Ahmed Datti.*

*(L-R)* ***Back****: Dr. Patrick Okao, Dr. Lawrence Sherman, Prof. Michael Kizza, Dr. Gue Atem, and Prof. Vuyu Kanda Golakai*

*Graduates of the first cohort – (Surgery) (L-R) Dr. Moses Fallah, Dr. Soliman Konneh. Dr. Terseer Utam, and Dr. Sengbe Vanyabah*

**FACULTY OF SURGERY GRADUATES**

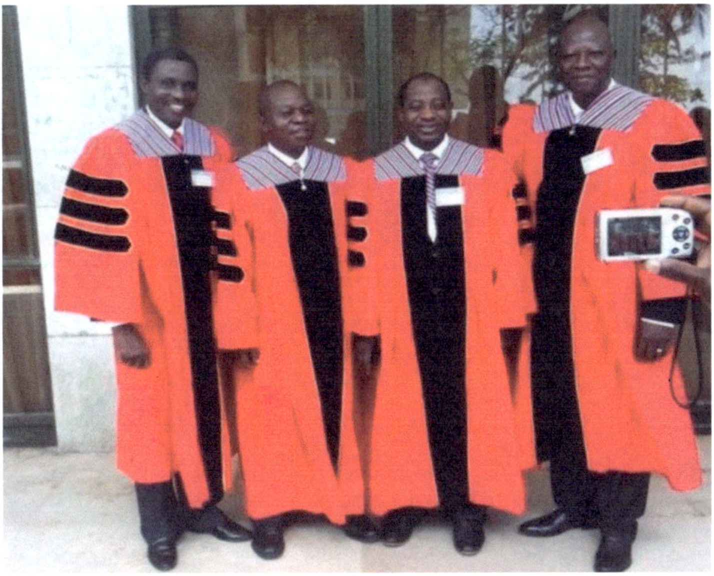

*L-R: Dr. Terseer Utam, Dr. Sengbe Vanyabah, Dr. Solimann Konneh & Dr. Moses Fallah*

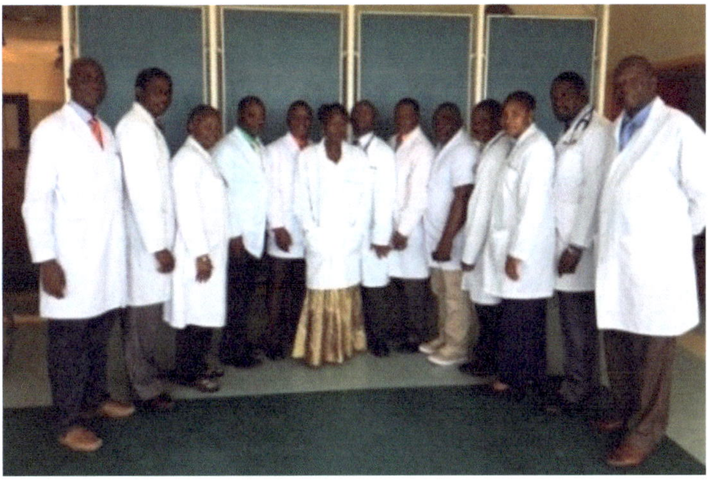

*All the First Graduands, LCPS 2017 (Surgeons & Physicians)*

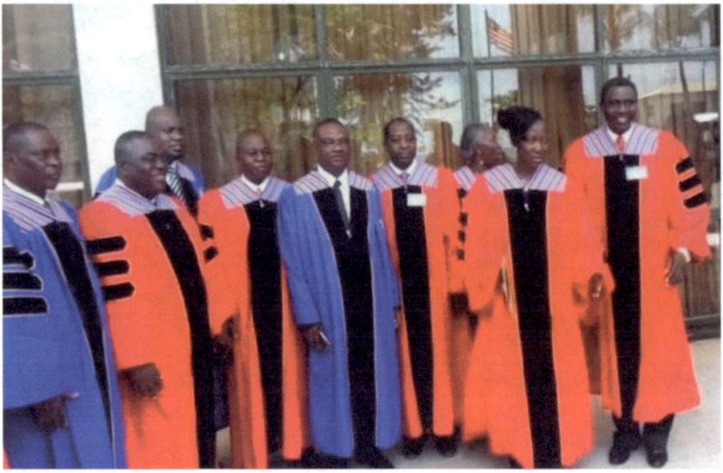

*The First (2017) graduation ceremony of LCPS*

In furtherance of LCPS fellowship program, the college on the 30th September 2022, at its 6th AGSM CONFERENCE, awarded 13 fellowships (12 by election and 1 honorary) to highly qualified faculty consultants and professors, plus one, to a great contributor to the development of psychiatry in the college.

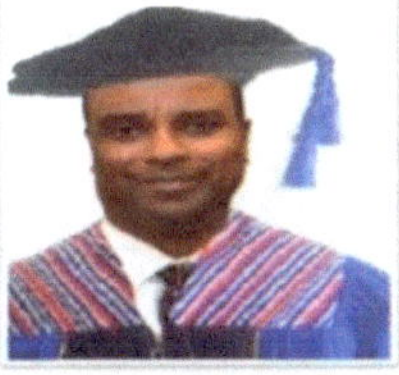

***Prof. David C. Henderson***
Honorary Fellow (Faculty of Psychiatry)

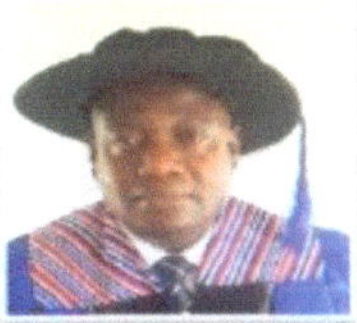

***Dr. Ian Wacheka***
Faculty of Internal Medicine

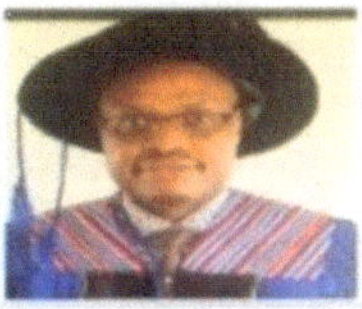

***Dr. Muhammad Awwal Abdullah***
Faculty of Internal Medicine

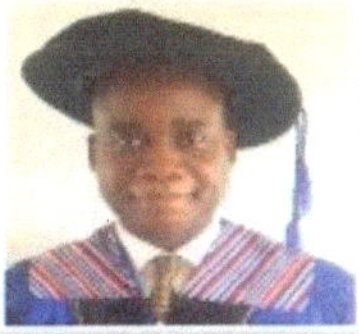

***Dr. Philip Z. Ireland***
Faculty of Internal Medicine

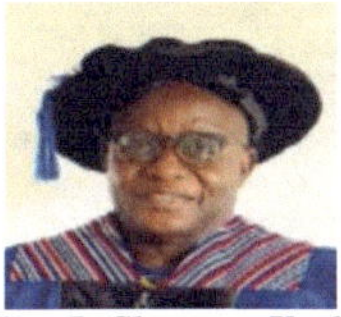

***Dr. J. Clarence Yaskey***
Faculty of Community Medicine

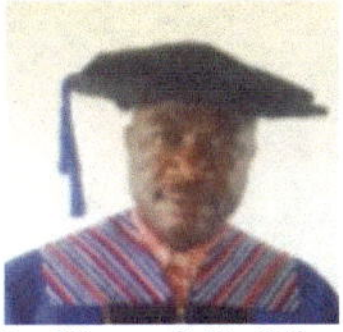

***Dr. Nnamdi E. Ojimadu***
Faculty of Family Medicine

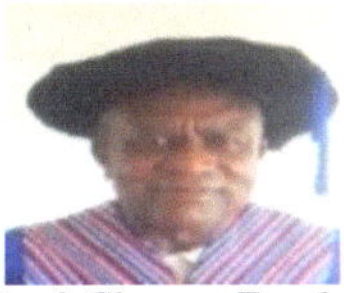

***Prof. Clement Ezechukwu***
Faculty of Pediatrics

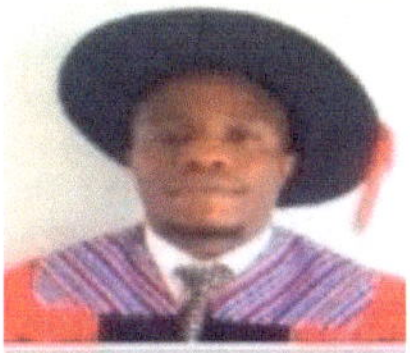

***Dr. Aaron H. Kokulol***
Faculty of Surgery

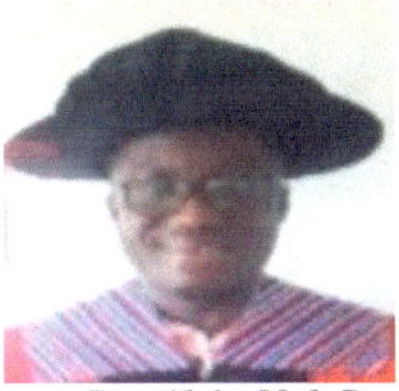

***Dr. Alvin Nah Doe***
Faculty of Surgery

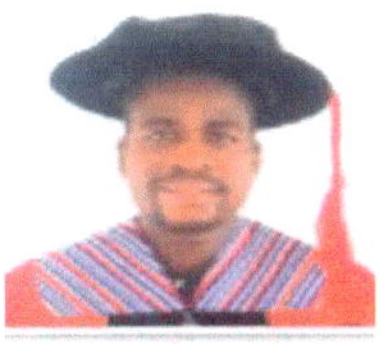

***Dr. Ayun K. Cassell***
Faculty of Surgery

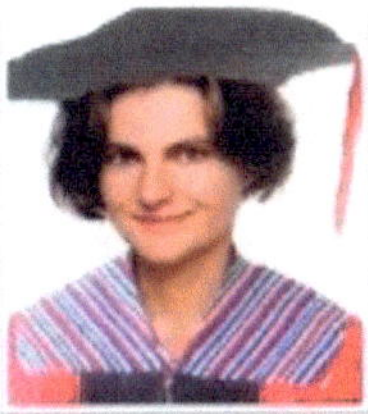

***Dr. Katja Maschuw***
Faculty of Surgery.

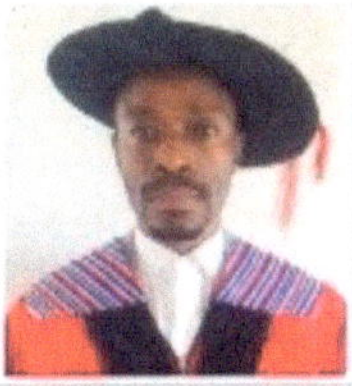

***Dr. Mabanza K. Tresor***
Faculty of Surgery.

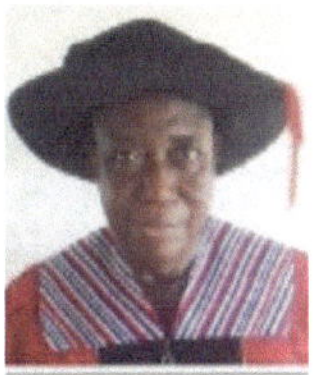

***Dr. Robert G. Mulbah***
Faculty of Surgery.

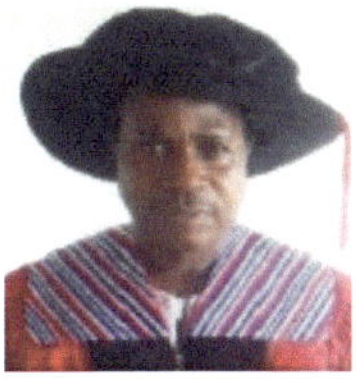

***Prof, Thomas U. Agan***
Faculty of Surgery

***EJS Ministerial Conference Center, Congo Town, Monrovia***

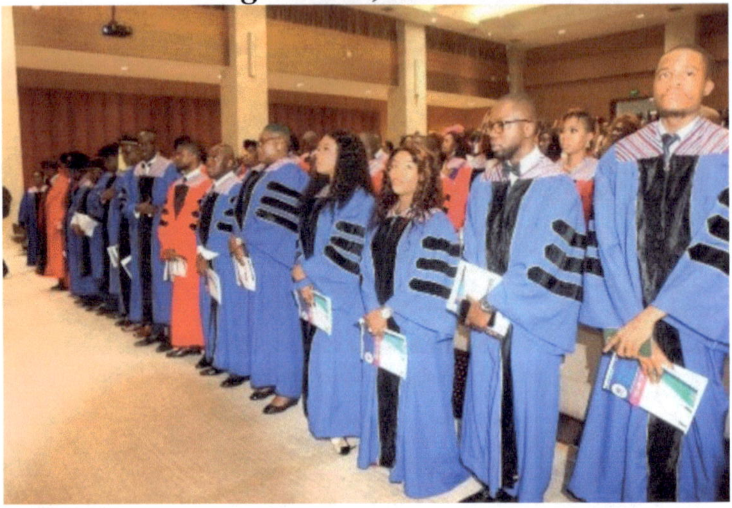

*LCPS 2022 Convocation*

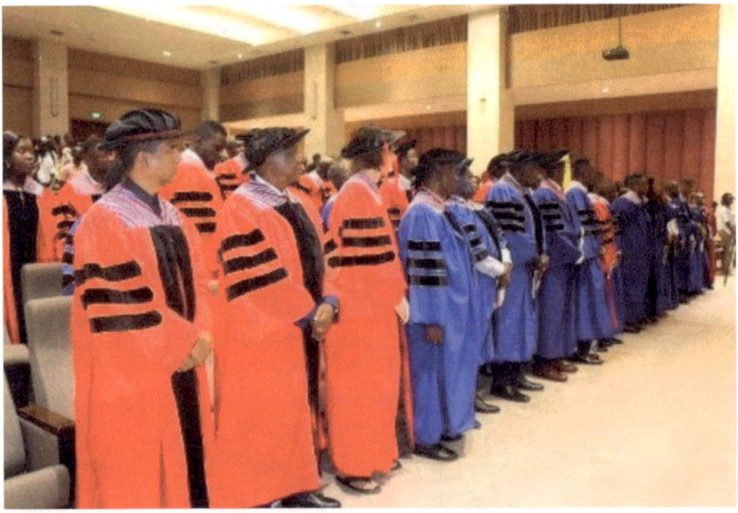

*Graduating Fellowship and membership*

# Chapter 9

## The Establishment of the Liberia Medical and Dental Council (LMDC)

### THE LIBERIA MEDICAL AND DENTAL COUNCIL

All the countries in the world that have healthcare delivery systems, training institutions, and medical practitioners do have instruments to regulate and monitor their activities.

Therefore, in the constitution of Liberia was enacted in 1967, a public health law that included a health regulatory body called the **Liberia Medical Board** which was controlled exclusively by the Ministry of Health. Among its functions were to regulate the establishment of health care and training institutions, their functions and licensure of health care practitioners.

Over the years, there occurred the need to amend and revise the Act, to accommodate the current realities. Therefore, the 1967 Health Act that created the Liberia Medical Board was revised in 2012 by an Act of legislature that did not only replace the Board with the **Liberia Medical and Dental Council** but also made **the new body autonomous to be headed by a medical doctor**.

Prior to this time the Medical Board was headed and controlled by successive Ministers of Health, who were not only political appointees but on many occasions were non-medical doctors charged with the responsibility to license doctors and health care service institutions.

This misnomer resulted into the mushrooming of established substandard healthcare institutions, and licensing of unqualified and even fake and bogus medical practitioners.

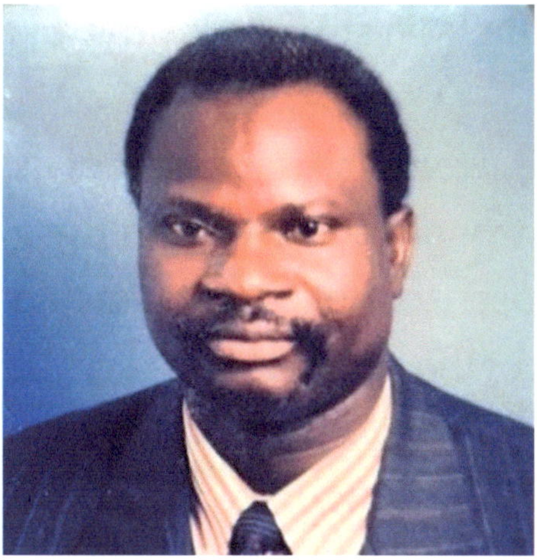

*Dr. Ivan Camanor*

It was not until 1985 when Dr. Ivan Camanor, former Chief Medical Officer/Deputy Minister of Health, established an Examination and Credentials Committee of the Medical Board and appointed me (Dr. Robert M. Kpoto) just returned from studies in England as its first chairman, that an enforcing regulatory body was actualized.

Together we established a system of assessment by clinical interviews, and written examinations of foreign trained doctors, coming in country. I set up the first separate Liberia Medical Board office at the old Maternity Center building on Capitol Bye- Pass in 1985. At the time the Ministry of Health was located in Sinkor.

Unfortunately, the tentacles of government were so strongly embedded in the system that it continued to put stumbling blocks to the functions of the committee.

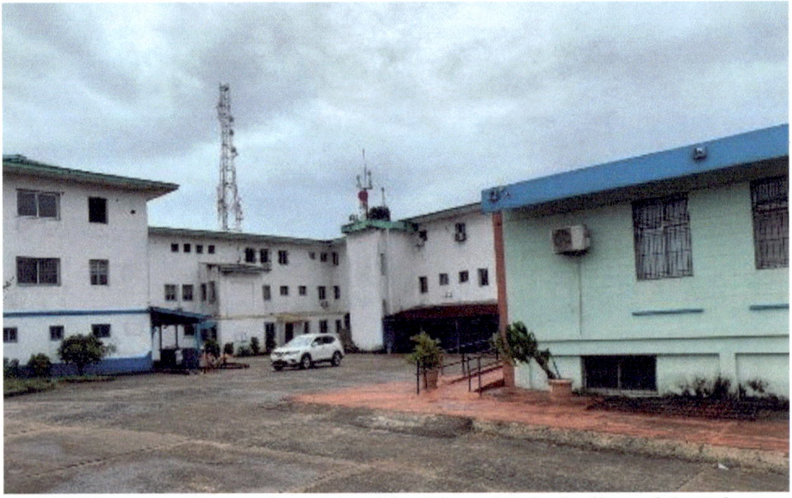

*Old Maternity Center, location of the 1st established office of the Liberia Medical Board*

In one graphic episode, an expatriate doctor was assessed by the Medical Board, found incompetent and therefore denied license to practice medicine in Liberia. His host and employer protested and appealed to the Liberian President who instructed his Minister of Health to grant the doctor license to practice.

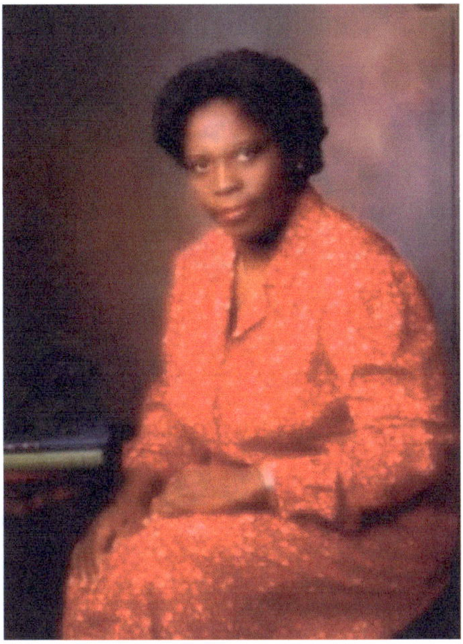

*Madam Martha Sandolo Belleh*
*Minister of Health*

The Minister, Madam Martha Sandolo Belleh who was a skilled professional administrator, upheld the Board's decision. Notwithstanding conveyed the President's message to the Chief Medical Officer and onto the committee. The President's request was rejected and the Board sustained its decision not to license the doctor.

The President in his anger said "then I qualify the doctor" and he immediately assigned him up country to practice without license.

That early incidence kindled my burning desire to fight for the Liberia Medical Board to become autonomous and independent of the Ministry of Health. That desire hibernated until 1992 when I was elected President of the Liberia Medical and Dental Association (LMDA).

Upon taking office, I immediately started a vehement campaign among law makers in the corridors of Capitol Hill to amend the Act that established the Board to make it independent of the Ministry of Health.

Twice, I introduced the bill in the Legislature and twice it was defeated. The sitting

Minister of Health engineered these defeats. He lobbied young doctors and highlighted a clause in the bill which stated that **after internship, doctors should sit an assessment exam before licensure.**

Their argument was that the need for an examination as a prerequisite for post internship licensure was redundant, since the examiners were the same lecturers that trained and qualified them to graduate.

Despite the defeats of the bills, I remained resolute and convinced that the proposed medical board did not only need to be autonomous, but to be expanded to a council with greater powers.

Fortunately, in 2000, I was elected Chairman of the Medical Board, and during my tenure, I encountered the relentless challenge from the Ministry resisting the autonomy of the Board.

These stumbling blocks opened room for the establishment of the **fake St. Luke School of Medicine** by some foreigners.

Unfortunately for the proprietor, fake diplomas given to some Indian "doctors" (copy below) landed in the hands of the Indian Consular, Upjit Singh Sachdeva ("Jetty"), who sent it to the Medical Board (I now head as Chairman) for verification and authentication.

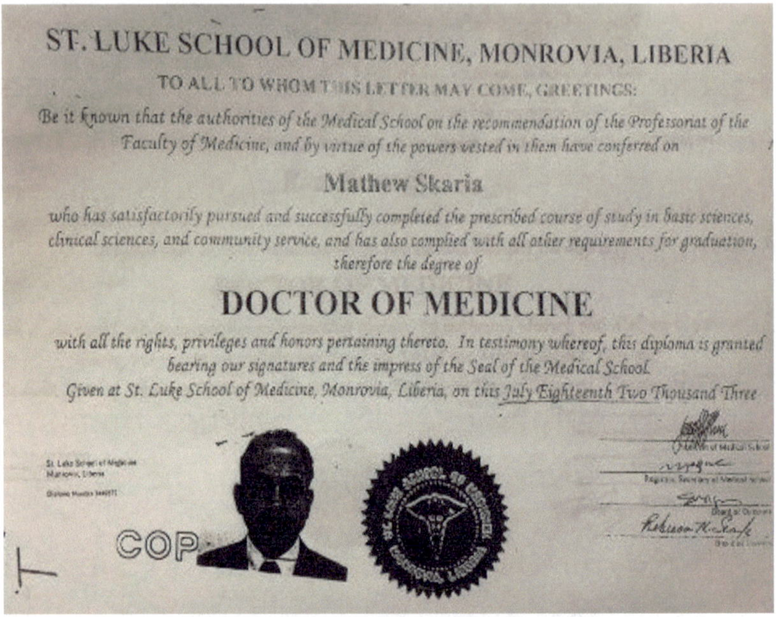

ST. LUKE SCHOOL OF MEDICINE, MONROVIA, LIBERIA

TO ALL TO WHOM THIS LETTER MAY COME, GREETINGS:

Be it known that the authorities of the Medical School on the recommendation of the Professoriat of the Faculty of Medicine, and by virtue of the powers vested in them have conferred on

Mathew Skaria

who has satisfactorily pursued and successfully completed the prescribed course of study in basic sciences, clinical sciences, and community service, and has also complied with all other requirements for graduation, therefore the degree of

DOCTOR OF MEDICINE

with all the rights, privileges and honors pertaining thereto. In testimony whereof, this diploma is granted bearing our signatures and the impress of the Seal of the Medical School.

Given at St. Luke School of Medicine, Monrovia, Liberia, on this July Eighteenth Two Thousand Three

COP

***Copy of fake diploma***

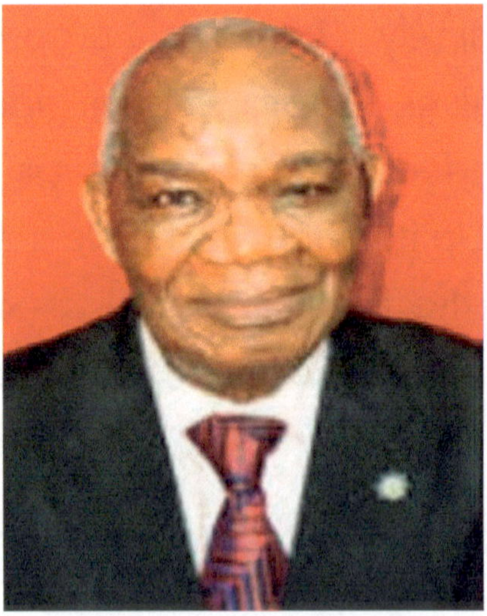

***Prof. S. Benson Barh***

I immediately mobilized support from Prof. Benson Barh, Deputy Minister of Health/CMO and Secretary General of the Board (He was also the 1st graduate of the college to become Dean of the institution).

On my team also was, Dr. S. Mohammed Sheriff, Chairman of the Standing Committee on health at the Legislature, and together we took legal action that closed the St. Luke School of Medicine.

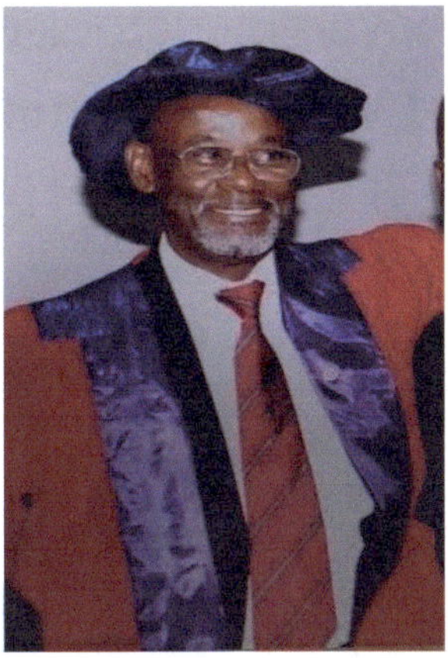

***Dr. S. Mohammed Sheriff***

Dr. Sheriff in subsequent years also held many cabinet and diplomatic portfolios that he levied to attract funding from the Italian government and other international institutions for developmental projects of the college.

After the closure of the St. Luke School of Medicine, I immediately transferred the office of the Board from the Ministry of Health building to its present premises hosting the LMDA on the JFK Compound.

From this new office I continued to pursue the autonomy process in collaboration, this time, with Executives of LMDA while at the same time praying for a change innational leadership to one that would welcome the pursuit for autonomy. By fortune, a new government took over the country and Dr. Walter Gwenigale, commonly called Dr. G, was appointed Minister of Health and Social Welfare.

Dr. G's selflessness and humble **willingness to relinquish his ministerial power and grip on the Liberia Medical Board**, and to give unconditional support, for the autonomy of the institution was unsurprisingly the coup de grace that finally removed the major stumbling block and permitted the passing of the bill that replaced the Liberia Medical Board with the **Liberia Medical and Dental Council (LMDC).**

At the same time, the Act made the council autonomous. I remembered Dr. G saying to the lawmakers during the legislative hearing at the Capitol Building to defend the bill.

> **"I don't need that power, and not any Minister of Health after me needs that power. Let the doctors be free to license themselves"** he, as usual, yelling to the law makers concluded.

That magnanimous, memorable statement as well as the singular bold decision by a sitting Minster of Health, unshackled the hands of the legislators to reconsider and revise the 1967 Act; thus, changing the Liberian Medical Board to the Liberia Medical and Dental Council.

Also, I invited for support at that hearing Dr. Taylor Neal (immediate past Chairman of the Board), Dr. Lynden Mabande, (immediate past President of LMDA), Dr. Moses Massaquoi, President of LMDA and Mrs. Morris, (Chairman of the Nursing Board).

Subsequently, on the 25th of March 2010, President Ellen Johnson Sirleaf signed the bill into law and on April 14, 2010, it was printed into Hand Bills. Thus, legally creating LMDC. At the council's first meeting, I was elected its first chairman. (See appendix 6 for other members).

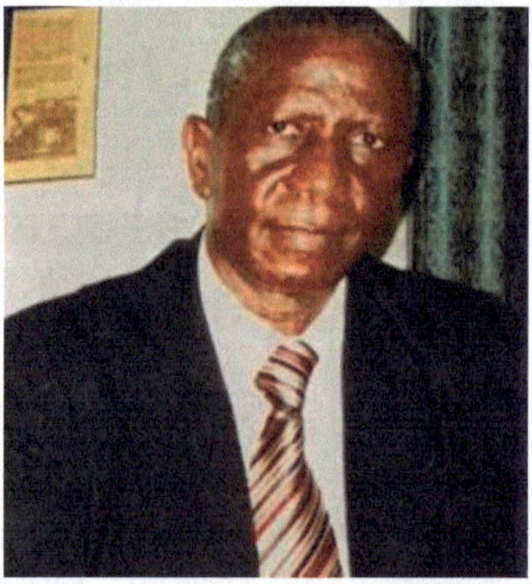

***1st Chairman LMDC/Prof. Robert M. Kpoto***

My first major task was to have the new council included in the national budget and to rehabilitate the new office. Along with LMDA executives, we lobbied for additional support from the Global Fund that helped to re-roof the building and put tiles in the conference room.

Following that, I put in personal financing pro-bono was able to complete the remaining rehabilitation and renovation of the LMDC & LMDA offices.

The additional renovation process included cutting down mango trees from the yard, building fence, digging septic tank, plumbing, electrification, carpentry (doors, ceilings), changing windows to sliding glasses, laying tiles in all the offices, building generator room, and buying a new generator, painting, air conditioner, curtains, new desks and chairs, internet system and computers.

I organized a complete financial management system, opened additional bank accounts, and set up a Government of Liberia (GoL) Tax Registry for LMDC among many more.

Since then, the Liberia Medical and Dental Council has become an indispensable, pivotal pillar in the operation of the National Health Care delivery system of the country.

It licenses doctors, health care and training institutions, regulates, conducts workshops, training, monitors, and in partnership with the Ministry of Health, advises on Health Polices, Decisions and Programs, among other functions.

# Section Four

LMDA: AN OVERVIEW

# Chapter 10

## A Brief History Of LMDA

The Liberia Medical and Dental Association (LMDA) was established in November of 1963 as the Liberia Medical Association (LMA) with Dr. Joseph Nagbe Togba as first President.

The association was established to serve as a forum for the exchange of ideas among members of the medical profession and in the allied sciences both Nationally and Internationally. To act as the National representative body for the Medical Profession as well as promote health care delivery in

Liberia. Additionally, the LMDA was to create a forum which will register all Medical Doctors in the Republic.

In 1970 the Dentists joined as members of the LMA, thus necessitating the change of name from LMA to LMDA.

Vision, Aims & Objectives

- To create a forum which will gather all medical doctors and dentists registered in Liberia
- To promote and maintain A high standard of professional practice, ethnics, dignity, and morals of medical doctors and dentists in Liberia
- To serve as a forum for the allied sciences both nationally and internationally.
- Dissemination of information and advice on health matters in Liberia.
- To promote health care delivery in Liberia
- To improve the welfare of the members
- To solicit support and engage in charitable activities
- To conduct research independently or in collaboration with the Ministry of Health and Social Welfare.

Over the years, the LMDA has had twenty (20) presidents, three of whom were females and three were expatriates. Today the LMDA continues to uphold its core aims and remains relevant to the medical community and the Republic.

## LIST OF PRESIDENTS OF LMA/LMDA UP TO 2022

1. Dr. Joseph N. Togba MD, MPH, FWACP (1963)
2. Dr. Nehemiah Cooper MD, FACS, FICS, FWACS
3. Dr. Kate Bryant MD, DCH, FWACP
4. Dr. Edwin Jallah MD, FACS, FACS
5. Dr. Charles Jupiter DDS
6. Dr. Varsay E Sirleaf MD, DTM, FWACP
7. Prof. Walter Brumskine MD, FRCS, FWACP
8. Dr. Walter Gwenigale MD, FLCPS
9. Dr. Wilfred Boayue MD, MPH, FWACP, FLCPS
10. Dr. Emile T. Woods MD
11. Dr. Bankole Jarrett MD, FWACP, FLCPS
12. Prof. Samuel V. Freeman MD, FRCS, FWACS, FLCPS
13. Dr. Nathaniel S. Bartee MD FLCPS
14. Prof. Robert M. Kpoto MD, FRCS, MCh (Ortho), FWACS, FLCPS
15. Dr. Lilly Sanvee MD, FLCPS
16. Dr. S. Benson Barh MD, MPH, FWACP, FLCPS
17. Dr. Eugene D. Dolopei MD, MPH, FWACP, FLCPS
18. Dr. Lyndon G.Mabande MD, PGDip, MPH, DLSHTM, FLCP
19. Dr. Moses Massaquoi MD, MPH, FWACP, FLCP
20. Dr. Louise M. Kpoto MD, MMED, MPH, PHD
21. Dr. Emmanuel Ekyanabah MD, MLCPS, FWACP
22. Dr. (Major) Albertha Clarke- Kollie (2022)

# Appendix I

## THE HIPPOCRATIC OATH: MODERN VERSION

I swear to fulfill, to the best of my ability and judgment, this covenant:

I will respect the hard-won scientific gains of those physicians in whose steps I walk, and gladly share such knowledge as is mine with those who are to follow.

I will apply, for the benefit of the sick, all measures [that] are required, avoiding those twin traps of overtreatment and therapeutic nihilism.

I will remember that there is art to medicine as well as science, and that warmth, sympathy, and understanding may outweigh the surgeon's knife or the chemist's drug.

I will not be ashamed to say "I know not," nor will I fail to call in my colleagues when the skills of another are needed for a patient's recovery.

I will respect the privacy of my patients, for their problems are not disclosed to me that the world may know. Most especially must I tread with care in matters of life and death. If it is given me to save a life, all thanks. But it may also be within my power to take a life; this awesome responsibility must be faced with great humbleness and awareness of my own frailty. Above all, I must not play at God.

I will remember that I do not treat a fever chart, a cancerous growth, but a sick human being, whose illness may affect the person's family and economic stability. My responsibility includes these related problems, if I am to care adequately for the sick.

I will prevent disease whenever I can, for prevention is preferable to cure.

I will remember that I remain a member of society, with special obligations to all my fellow human beings, those sound of mind and body as well as the infirm.

If I do not violate this oath, may I enjoy life and art, respected while I live and remembered with affection thereafter. May I always act so as to preserve the finest traditions of my calling and may I long experience the joy of healing those who seek my help.

# Appendix 2

## Historical Highlights of the A.M. Dogliotti College of Medicine

- President William V. S. Tubman conceived the vision for Liberia to train its own medical doctors sometimes in the early to mid-1950's [1956-1964]

- Mobilization of Technical and Financial Support for the establishment of a medical school in Liberia was a joint venture involving the Governments of Liberia and Italy, as wells as the Holy See (Vatican) and the Dogliotti Foundation during the period of 1964-1966. The agreement between the Italian Government and the A.M. Dogliotti Foundation to support the establishment of the medical school in Liberia was finalized in 1966.
- Since the Italian academic institution that was assigned the task of developing and implementing the curriculum of the medical school in Monrovia, Liberia was the University of Torino located in the city of Torino, the new medical school was named the Monrovia-Torino College of Medicine.

This Monrovia-Torino College of Medicine in Liberia was affiliated with the Faculty of Medicine and Surgery of the University of Torino.

- Groundbreaking ceremony for the construction of the Monrovia-Torino College of Medicine was done in 1966 in Congo Town, Monrovia, Liberia. President William V. S. Tubman represented the government of Liberia, Archbishop Francis Carroll represented the Holy See (Vatican) and the Italian Ambassador accredited near Monrovia represented the Italian government.
- The original campus of the medical school included an academic building, a teaching hospital (currently the Catholic Hospital), a dormitory and an administrative building.
- While the campus of the medical school was under construction, the two-year pre-medical program of the college started on the campus of the St. Patrick High School in Monrovia in March of 1966.
- In 1967, the Monrovia-Torino Medical College facilities were formally inaugurated. During this same year, the pre-medical program of the Monrovia- Torino College of Medicine was incorporated into the science college curriculum of the University of Liberia.
- In 1968, The Monrovia-Torino College of Medicine admitted its first set of first year medical students.
- In 1970 the Monrovia-Torino College of Medicine was merged with the University of Liberia as the seventh academic program, and the second professional school (the Law School being the first professional school).

At this same time the college was renamed the Achille Mario Dogliotti College of Medicine, after the late Italian philanthropist and founder of the Dogliotti Foundation in Italy.

- In 1971, the John F. Kennedy Memorial Hospital was inaugurated and became the teaching hospital of the A. M. Dogliotti College of Medicine. The first class of medical students entered the clinical program of the medical college at the John F. Kennedy Memorial Hospital in July 1971.

- In December 1973, the A. M. Dogliotti College of Medicine graduated its first set of medical students with the degree of Doctor of Medicine (MD).

- In 1983, the A. M. Dogliotti College of Medicine reached a milestone with the graduation of its first 100th medical doctor when 16 students graduated in that year.

- The support of the Italian government and the Dogliotti Foundation was scaled down according to plan in the 1980's before the inception of the 14- year civil war of Liberia which started in December 1989. The Liberian civil war adversely affected every aspect of the medical college program to the point that the institution was automatically closed in May 1990 and then reopened with the bare minimum training capacity in 1992. After the re- opening, the World Health Organization (WHO) and the Roman Catholic Church of Liberia were the major supporting organizations of the medical college.

# Appendix 3

## Roster of Graduates (AMDC)

### A.M. Dogliotti College of Medicine (1973 – 2022)

| No. NAME | Gender | COUNTY/COUNTRY |
|---|---|---|
| **December 11, 1973** | | |
| 1. Bowman, Samuel | M | Maryland (Liberia) |
| 2. Izundu, Micheal | M | Nigeria |
| 3. Kurien, Susamma | F | India |
| 4. Seton, Moses | M | Nigeria |
| **December 10, 1974** | | |
| 5. Adams, Z'sherman | M | Grand Bassa (Liberia) |
| 6. Agu, Chuke | M | Nigeria |
| 7. Dafiluelo, Clemet | M | Nigeria |
| 8. Kpoto, Robert | M | Lofa (Liberia) |
| 9. Lewis, Emmanuel Kai | M | Sinoe (Liberia) |
| 10. Metieh, Paul | M | Nigeria |
| 11. Okonkwo, Albert | M | Nigeria |
| 12. Okonmah, Augustine | M | Nigeria |
| 13. Okoye, Ambrose | M | Nigeria |
| 14. Afolabi Oyelayo, Oyesola | M | Nigeria |
| **December 12, 1975** | | |
| 15. Abayomi-Cole, Alfred | M | Sierra Leone |
| 16. Akanji, Ademola | M | Nigeria |
| 17. Anumba, Sylvester | M | Nigeria |
| 18. Deciman, Ring | M | Sudan |
| 19. Dennis, Josephine | F | Liberia |

| | | |
|---|---|---|
| 20. Devine, Patricia | F | Liberia |
| 21. Ezeamah, Felix | M | Nigeria |
| 22. Komeh, Edward | M | Sierra Leone |
| 23. Njoh, Joseph | M | Nigeria |
| 24. Osibo, Akinrinola | M | Nigeria |
| 25. Sankoh, Mohammed | M | Sierra Leone |
| 26. Sasaraku, Samuel | M | Ghana |

**1976**

| | | |
|---|---|---|
| 27. Adeyera, Amos A. | M | Nigeria |
| 28. Carmanor, Ivan B. | M | Lofa (Liberia) |
| 29. Chellaram, Ram | M | India |
| 30. Galakpai, Moses K. | M | Lofa (Liberia) |
| 31. Viddy, Antonio | M | Angola |

**December 14, 1977**

| | | |
|---|---|---|
| 32. Ajose, Anthony O. | M | Nigeria |
| 33. Barclay, Emmanuel | M | Liberia |
| 34. Harris, Benjamin | M | Liberia |
| 35. Opawoye, Adebayo | M | Nigeria |
| 36. Reeves, Henry | M | Liberia |
| 37. Swaray, Mustapha | M | Liberia |

**December 13, 1978**

| | | |
|---|---|---|
| 38. Amable, Eugene | M | Ghana |
| 39. Barh, S. Benson | M | Grand Gedeh |
| 40. Findley, Alfonso C. | M | Grand Bassa |
| 41. Jallah, Karsor J. | M | Lofa (Liberia) |
| 42. Madut, Buok | M | Sudan |
| 43. Mzezewa, Salathiel | M | Rhodesia |
| 44. Benson, Jimi O. | M | Nigeria |
| 45. Omolokun, Omobola | M | Nigeria |
| 46. Nicolas, Pierre P. | M | Haiti |
| 47. Webba, Joao V. | M | Angola |
| 48. White, Albert T. Jr. | M | Montserrado |

**December 18, 1979**

| | | |
|---|---|---|
| 49. Amadi, Ngeri | F | Nigeria |
| 50. Avorkliyah, Julius | M | Liberia |
| 51. Jalloh, Idriss Francis | M | Sierra Leone |
| 52. Jalloh, Ibrahim | M | Sierra Leone |
| 53. Kanneh, Mohammed Vamba. | M | Lofa (Liberia) |
| 54. Kolawole, Titus | M | Nigeria |
| 55. Major, Velma | F | Liberia |
| 56. Pedro, Angelo | M | Angola |
| 57. Railey, Yvonne | F | Liberia |
| 58. Waiwaiku, Kokulo | M | Lofa (Liberia) |

**1980**

| | | |
|---|---|---|
| 59. Amet-Simbeye, Isabella | F | Liberia |
| 60. Boayue, Yao Tonieh | F | Nimba (Liberia) |
| 61. Browne, Isaac | M | Sinoe (Liberia) |
| 62. Carew, Kojo | M | Sierra Leone |
| 63. Diggs, Margaret | F | Liberia |
| 64. Ekanem-Thompson, Donald | M | Nigeria |
| 65. Findley, Gertrude | F | Liberia |
| 66. Jallah, Rose | F | Lofa (Liberia) |
| 67. Maximore, Sara | F | Liberia |
| 68. Muctarr, Khadijatu | F | Liberia |
| 69. Ndamse, Richard S. | M | South Africa |
| 70. Nimley, Victoria | F | Sinoe (Liberia) |
| 71. Onyekwum, Allison | M | Nigeria |
| 72. Parwon, Sie-M II | M | Nimba (Liberia) |
| 73. Pieh, Michael | M | Liberia |
| 74. Shaw, Alfred Eddie | M | Liberia |
| 75. Sidile, Eric | M | Rhodesia |
| 76. Takyi, Frank Kwasi | M | Ghana |
| 77. Uchendu, Catherine | F | Nigeria |
| 78. Wolo, Mac-Arthur | M | Liberia |

**December 16, 1981**

| | | |
|---|---|---|
| 79. Awode, Cecelia C. | F | Montserrado |
| 80. Bartee, Nathaniel S. | M | Sinoe (Liberia) |
| 81. Flahn, G. Ninneh | M | Grand Gedeh |
| 82. Freeman, Tabeh L. | M | Maryland |
| 83. George, Raju Jacob | M | India |
| 84. Igwe, Gene Wilson | M | Nigeria |
| 85. Jones, Michael A. | M | Bong (Liberia) |
| 86. Kiawoin, Kedrick K. | M | Cape Mount |
| 87. Makakole, Lipontso | F | Lesotho |
| 88. Mends-Cole, Corrine | F | Montserrado |
| 89. Musa, Sele B. | M | Lofa (Liberia) |
| 90. Ndamse, Jennifer | F | South Africa |
| 91. Ndlovu, Austin | M | Zimbabwe |
| 92. Ngere, Paul M. | M | Zimbabwe |
| 93. Nicolas, Guy E. | M | Montserrado |
| 94. Thomas, Francis H. | M | Bong (Liberia) |
| 95. Troko, D. Memba | M | Nimba (Liberia) |
| 96. Xerinda, Paulo E. | M | Mozambique |
| 97. Yuoh, Gbo | M | Nimba (Liberia) |

**February 16, 1983**

| | | |
|---|---|---|
| 98. Adekoya, Thomas O. | M | Montserrado |
| 99. Bah, Kadijatu | F | Sierra Leone |
| 100. Dakinah, Gbatokai F. | M | Montserrado |
| 101. Davies-Makwi, Glena O. | F | Sierra Leone |
| 102. Dukuly, Zwannah D. | M | Montserrado |
| 103. Elliotti, James W. | M | Grand Kru |
| 104. Harris, Wilmot S. W. | M | Bong (Liberia) |
| 105. Hove, Vushe J. | M | Zimbabwe |
| 106. Kamanda, William S. | M | Lofa (Liberia) |
| 107. Makwi, Kylkon | M | Bong (Liberia) |
| 108. Mayson, Robert P. | M | Sinoe (Liberia) |
| 109. Mensah, G. Tetteh | M | Montserrado |
| 110. Mwaipola, Whitson E. | M | Tanzania |
| 111. Njinimbam, Charles C. G. | M | Cameroon |
| 112. Sawyer, Valentine G. | M | Montserrado |
| 113. Zawu, Siba Kaly | M | Lofa (Liberia) |

**December 21, 1983**

| | | | |
|---|---|---|---|
| 114. | Amao, Akinwumi K. | M | Nigeria |
| 115. | Blegy, Robert N. | M | Nimba (Liberia) |
| 116. | Chirenje, Zvavhera | M | Rhodesia |
| 117. | Diallo, Alpha A. | M | Montserrado |
| 118. | Doe, Nathaniel S. | M | Montserrado |
| 119. | Doe, Pylord P. | M | Sinoe (Liberia) |
| 120. | Kouroma, Augustine | M | Montserrado |
| 121. | Olanipekun, Babatunde | M | Nigeria |
| 122. | Reeves, Inez Vera | F | Montserrado |
| 123. | Scott, Henrique Z. | M | Montserrado |
| 124. | Willicor, Albert G. | M | Lofa |

**April 24, 1985**

| | | | |
|---|---|---|---|
| 125. | Asase, Danilo Koku | M | Ghana |
| 126. | Darpolor, Joseph | M | Lofa (Liberia) |
| 127. | Freeman, Harrison | M | Maryland |
| 128. | French, Winifred | F | Sierra Leone |
| 129. | Gadegbeku, Patience | F | Grand Gedeh |
| 130. | Logan, Sabrina | F | Montserrado |
| 131. | Saah, Daniel T. | M | Lofa |

**May 7, 1986**

| | | | |
|---|---|---|---|
| 132. | Akena, Charles | M | Uganda |
| 133. | Boayu, Koh B. | M | Nimba (Liberia) |
| 134. | Croffie, Joseph | M | Ghana |
| 135. | George, Rani Elizabeth | F | India |
| 136. | Mabande, Lyndon G. | M | Cape Mount |
| 137. | Marbiah, Nuahn T. | M | Nimba (Liberia) |
| 138. | Musana, Andrew | M | Sierra Leone |
| 139. | Saab, Benedict | M | Grand Bassa |
| 140. | Sheriff, Momodu | M | Cape Mount |
| 141. | Sleweon, Thomas | M | Maryland |

**July 22, 1987**

| | | | |
|---|---|---|---|
| 142. | Barrolle, Vivian K. | F | Montserrado |
| 143. | Benson, Adongakulu O. | M | Uganda |
| 144. | Dennis, Tshekedi G. | M | Montserrado |
| 145. | Dolopei, Eugene D. | M | Nimba |
| 146. | Eben, Martin T. | M | Cameroon |
| 147. | Enchill, Richard K. | M | Ghana |
| 148. | Flomo, Korwan Z. | M | Lofa (Liberia) |
| 149. | Gbokolo, Kouneway G. | F | Nimba (Liberia) |
| 150. | Bettie, Harrison R. | M | Grand Bassa |
| 151. | Barclay, James K. | M | Bong (Liberia) |
| 152. | Johnson, Fayemi | M | Sierra Leone |
| 153. | Kear, Moses D. | M | Grand Gedeh |
| 154. | Konuwa, Henry A. | M | Cape Mount |
| 155. | Major, Maud O. | F | Montserrado |
| 156. | Daramy, Mohammed L. | M | Sierra Leone |
| 157. | Samura, Fasineh S. | M | Sierra Leone |
| 158. | Tamu, Sheku B. | M | Sierra Leone |
| 159. | Tarawali, Moses B. | M | Montserrado |
| 160. | Wilson-Agwu, Ndidiamaka | F | Sierra Leone |
| 161. | Wreh, Victoria | F | Grand Bassa |
| 162. | York, Serena | F | Montserrado |

**June 27, 1988**

| | | | |
|---|---|---|---|
| 163. | Bonar, Adolphus S. | M | Grand Bassa |
| 164. | Cooper-Merchant, Eugenia | F | Grand Gedeh |
| 165. | Fahnbulleh, Augustus | M | Cape Mount |
| 166. | Frimpong, Patrick | M | Montserrado |
| 167. | Hall, Alvin J. | M | Bong (Liberia) |
| 168. | Musa, Joseph P. | M | Lofa (Liberia) |
| 169. | Siafa, Samuel R. | M | Lofa (Liberia) |

**May 3, 1989**

| | | | |
|---|---|---|---|
| 170. | Amara, Patrick | M | Bomi (Liberia) |
| 171. | Annie, Frederick J. | M | Ghana |

| | | | |
|---|---|---|---|
| 172. | Barclay, Elizabeth | F | Montserrado |
| 173. | Bayagbona, Barbara | F | Nigeria |
| 174. | Conneh, Musu J. | M | Bong (Liberia) |
| 175. | Chukwunere, Emmanuel | M | Nigeria |
| 176. | Cooper, Comfort S. | F | Montserrado |
| 177. | Domah, Nau D. | F | Nimba (Liberia) |
| 178. | Gbadouway, Charles | M | River Cess |
| 179. | Harding, Yvonne | F | Sierra Leone |
| 180. | Johnson, Peterlyne | F | Grand Geded |
| 181. | Johnson, Alexander P. | M | Lofa (Liberia) |
| 182. | Kieh, Mark | M | Sinoe (Liberia) |
| 183. | Kennedy, Stephen | M | Bong (Liberia) |
| 184. | Lincoln, Adams K. | M | Maryland |
| 185. | Lloyd, Davidetta | F | Grand Bassa |
| 186. | Nimely, Contah S. | F | River Cess |
| 187. | Onanuga, Ibitola A. | M | Nigeria |
| 188. | Topor, Patrick | M | Montserrado |
| 189. | Vokpor, Samuel | M | Lofa (Liberia) |

**February 16, 1990**

| | | | |
|---|---|---|---|
| 190. | Dennis, Mark | M | Sierra Leone |
| 191. | Jallah, Matthias N. | F | Lofa (Liberia) |
| 192. | Johnson, Jeanetta K. | F | Montserrado |
| 193. | Kaba, Martin | M | Cameroon |
| 194. | Kargbo, Nyanquoi K. | M | Lofa (Liberia) |
| 195. | Massaquoi, Moses | M | Lofa (Liberia) |
| 196. | NIcolls, Kelvin | M | Sierra Leone |
| 197. | Snellborough, Wilhemina | F | Montserrado |
| 198. | Yaskey, John C. | M | Margibi |

**March 8, 1994**

| | | | |
|---|---|---|---|
| 199. | Amagashie, Fred W. | M | Margibi |
| 200. | Baawo, Saye Dahn | M | Nimba (Liberia) |
| 201. | Dada, Taban J. | M | Uganda |
| 202. | Duworko, James T. | M | Lofa (Liberia) |
| 203. | Saah, James A.K. | M | Lofa (Liberia) |

| | | | |
|---|---|---|---|
| 204. | Sherman, Lawrence M. | M | Montserrado |
| 205. | Sobboh, James A. | M | Sinoe (Liberia) |
| 206. | Wolo, Jestina F. | F | Montserrado |
| 207. | Gill, Parminder F. | F | India |

**September 25, 1996**

| | | | |
|---|---|---|---|
| 208. | Beh, Goffa C. | M | Grand Bassa |
| 209. | Brewer, Jimmi N. | M | Nimba (Liberia) |
| 210. | Hunter, Emmanuel | M | Liberia |
| 211. | Koboi, J. Gayflor | M | Lofa (Liberia) |
| 212. | Moses, J. Fallah | M | Lofa (Liberia) |
| 213. | Passewe, Boakai | M | Cape Mount |
| 214. | Punni, Nyeotti N. | M | Sinoe (Liberia) |
| 215. | Saytarton, Wilson | M | Sinoe (Liberia) |
| 216. | Sieh, Clementia K. | F | Grand Kru |
| 217. | Tamakloe, Bernice | F | Maryland |
| 218. | Tamba, John F. | M | Lofa (Liberia) |
| 219. | Vonhm, Benjamin T. | M | Nimba (Liberia) |
| 220. | Browne-Passewe, Dahlene K. | F | Bong (Liberia) |
| 221. | Jeuronlon, Moses K. | M | Bong (Liberia) |
| 222. | Kamara, Mohammed | M | Lofa (Liberia) |
| 223. | Sando, Emmanuel | M | Lofa (Liberia) |
| 224. | Stewart-Stubblefield, Charlotte | F | Montserrado |
| 225. | Williams, Garfee T. | M | Maryland |

**June 2, 1998**

| | | | |
|---|---|---|---|
| 226. | Moibah, Nathaniel J. | M | Liberia |
| 227. | Quayee, Anthony S. | M | Lofa (Liberia) |
| 228. | Borbor, Abraham S. | M | Lofa (Liberia) |
| 229. | Jones, Joel J. | M | Montserrado |
| 230. | Korboi, Tete N. | F | Lofa (Liberia) |
| 231. | Prall, Jemmah | M | Lofa (Liberia) |
| 232. | Braima, Tamba S. | M | Lofa (Liberia) |
| 233. | Dioubate, Mitchel A. | M | Montserrado |
| 234. | Howard, Hayford M. | M | Lofa (Liberia) |

| | | | |
|---|---|---|---|
| 235. | Mansalay, Abu B. | M | Montserrado |
| 236. | Pabs-Garnon, Ian B. | M | Sierra Leone |

**December 19, 2001**

| | | | |
|---|---|---|---|
| 237. | Boker, Roxanne B. | F | Montserrado |
| 238. | Doe, Martha N. | F | Nimba (Liberia) |
| 239. | Kromah, Raymond F. | M | Cape Mount |
| 240. | Pratt, Philderald E. | M | Grand Bassa |
| 241. | Sibley, Jefferson K. | M | Bong (Liberia) |
| 242. | Thomas, Catherine E. | F | Nimba (Liberia) |

**May 28, 2003**

| | | | |
|---|---|---|---|
| 243. | Birch, Linda A. | F | Sinoe (Liberia) |
| 244. | Brown, Jerry F. | M | Bong (Liberia) |
| 245. | Camara, Ansumana F. | M | Lofa (Liberia) |
| 246. | Ekyinbah, Emmanuel K. | M | Montserrado |
| 247. | Geu, Atem D. | M | Sudan |
| 248. | Jebbeh, Caullau L. | F | Maryland |
| 249. | Jayasuriya, Sebastian L. | M | Sri Lanka |
| 250. | Johnson, Nittie K. | F | Montserrado |
| 251. | Mapleh, Louise C. | F | Grand Bassa |
| 252. | Wesseh, Paul T. | M | Grand Bassa |
| 253. | Wollor, Benedict N. | M | Grand Kru |

**February 22, 2006**

| | | | |
|---|---|---|---|
| 254. | Arzoaquoi, Sampson K. | M | Lofa (Liberia) |
| 255. | Collins, Benetta W. | F | Maryland |
| 256. | Lewis, James N. | M | Sinoe (Liberia) |
| 257. | Moore, Hawa B. | F | Montserrado |
| 258. | Nuta, Cecelia J. | F | Nimba (Liberia) |
| 259. | Sieka, Joseph M. | M | Grand Kru |
| 260. | Toe-Massaquoi, Rosalyn | F | Grand Kru |

**April 4, 2007**

| | | | |
|---|---|---|---|
| 261. | Ballah, Ngormbu | M | Lofa (Liberia) |
| 262. | Frank Jr., Wilmot G. | M | Grand Bassa |
| 263. | Garbo, Julius Y. | M | Lofa (Liberia) |
| 264. | Geah, Kour E. | F | Nimba (Liberia) |
| 265. | George, Josiah T. | M | River Gee |
| 266. | Jallabah, Torsou Y. | M | Montserrado |
| 267. | Kollie, Aaron Y. | M | Lofa (Liberia) |
| 268. | Kumah, Odell W. | F | Grand Kru |
| 269. | Minah, Abu B. | M | Sierra Leone |
| 270. | Roberts, Rhoda N. | F | Nimba (Liberia) |
| 271. | Sahr, Philip K. | M | Lofa (Liberia) |
| 272. | Toomey, Julia H. | F | Maryland |
| 273. | Vanyanbah, Saygbeh M. | M | Lofa (Liberia) |

**April 29, 2009**

| | | | |
|---|---|---|---|
| 274. | Karbah, Doryea F. W. | M | Lofa (Liberia) |
| 275. | Korvieh, James K. | M | Lofa (Liberia) |
| 276. | Pajibo Jr., Myer Chea | M | Sinoe (Liberia) |
| 277. | Tucker, Anthony M. | M | Cape Mount |

**December 16, 2009**

| | | | |
|---|---|---|---|
| 278. | Bedell Jr., Charles Teba | M | Maryland |
| 279. | Bowah, Collins Saa | M | Lofa (Liberia) |
| 280. | Daboi, Esther Korpo | F | Lofa (Liberia) |
| 281. | Diggs, Wiyata Tamara | F | Cape Mount |
| 282. | Igwilo, Patrick O. | M | Montserrado |
| 283. | Jawara, Abraham | M | Montserrado |
| 284. | Karmbor, Elsie Gufa | F | Grand Kru |
| 285. | Keita, Abraham Nyuma | M | Lofa (Liberia) |
| 286. | Logan, Gorbee Gabriel | M | Grand Bassa |
| 287. | Mulbah, Robert Gayflor | M | Lofa (Liberia) |
| 288. | Sackie, Yatta Docious | F | Bong (Liberia) |
| 289. | Smith, Wilmot Lorenzo | M | Sinoe (Liberia) |
| 290. | Washington, Trokon T. | M | Grand Bassa |

**May 4, 2011**

| | | | |
|---|---|---|---|
| 291. | Bolongei, Josephus Ernest. | M | Bong (Liberia) |
| 292. | Cooper, Lorraine C. | F | Montserrado |
| 293. | Doedeh Jr., John S. | M | Rivercess |
| 294. | Gayedyu, Dehkontee L. | F | Grand Bassa |
| 295. | Ireland, Philip Z. | M | Maryland |
| 296. | Kanagasabai, Udhayashankar | M | Sri Lanka |
| 297. | Kawah, Maima D. | F | Cape Mount |
| 298. | Mayah, Finda S. | F | Lofa (Liberia) |
| 299. | Moses, J. Soka | M | Lofa (Liberia) |
| 300. | Okwumuo, Celina M. | F | Rivercess |
| 301. | Tennih, Kormassa S. | F | Lofa (Liberia) |
| 302. | Williams, Williametta S. | F | Maryland |
| 303. | Yeiah, Adolphus T. | M | Nimba (Liberia) |

**May 9, 2012**

| | | | |
|---|---|---|---|
| 304. | Brima, Annette M. | F | Lofa |
| 305. | Catakaw, Kollie D. | M | Lofa |
| 306. | Dadzie, Jeffrey Eugene | M | Margibi |
| 307. | Freeman Jr., Tabeh L. | M | Maryland |
| 308. | Gayflor, Joseph | M | Lofa (Liberia) |
| 309. | Gbanlon, Nutia K. | F | Nimba (Liberia) |
| 310. | Gbanmie, Paye Nelson | F | Nimba (Liberia) |
| 311. | Gobeh Jr., Alan S. | M | Lofa (Liberia) |
| 312. | Hessou, Flinhway | F | Grand Kru |
| 313. | Kaman, Vanyah C. | F | Gbarpolu |
| 314. | Kortimai Jr., Lavela B. | M | Lofa (Liberia) |
| 315. | Kparteh, Zoebon B. | M | Montserrado |
| 316. | Kumblytee, Lawuobahsumo | F | Lofa (Liberia) |
| 317. | Nelson, Thelma Veronica | F | Montserrado |
| 318. | Nuahn, Gonkarnue | M | Nimba (Liberia) |
| 319. | Sankoh, Sovich Chica | F | Maryland |
| 320. | Barclay, Yassah M. | F | Lofa |
| 321. | Bartekwa, Joyce W. | F | Grand Kru |
| 322. | Benson, Williefrank A | M | Bong |

| | | |
|---|---|---|
| 323. Cassell, III, Ayun K | M | Bong |
| 324. Collins, Moretti Pah | M | River Gee |
| 325. Dono, Patience C | F | Cape Mount |
| 326. Dorbor, Korto T. | F | Lofa |
| 327. Duyenku, Fokape B | M | Lofa |
| 328. Enders, Numeine Ernest | M | Gbarpolu |
| 329. Fahnbulleh, II., L-Momoh G. | M | Cape Mount |
| 330. Fannieh, Augustine N. | M | Grand Kru |
| 331. Gbozee, Lawuobah | M | Lofa |
| 332. George, Methodius Taone | M | Maryland |
| 333. Gilayeneh, Julius S.M. | M | Nimba |
| 334. Goyah, Kezelebah S. | M | Lofa |
| 335. Gray, Keith Lancedall | M | Maryland |
| 336. Gwaikolo, Cozie | M | Nimba |
| 337. Harmon, Wahdae-Mai | F | Maryland |
| 338. Harris, Solomon Vomo | M | Lofa Liberia |
| 339. Hart, Jonathan M. | M | Montserrado |
| 340. Jetoh, Ralph W. | M | Sinoe Liberia |
| 341. Kamara, Patrick Lahai | M | Montserrado |
| 342. King, Detoh T | M | River Cess |
| 343. Kokulol, Aaron Hoto | M | Lofa Liberia |
| 344. Korheina, Levi D | M | Lofa Liberia |
| 345. Kumbuyah, Lucretia Siah | F | Lofa |
| 346. Massaley, Momolu | M | Cape Mount |
| 347. Nemah, Yuah A. | M | Maryland |
| 348. Saywon, Deazee M | M | Nimba Liberia |
| 349. Scotland, Jr., Thomas S. | M | River Cess |
| 350. Sesay, Claresia K | F | Bong Liberia |
| 351. Sheriff, Swaliho M. | M | Lofa Liberia |
| 352. Sonii, Hawa Adoley | F | Cape Mount |
| 353. Tehmeh, Lekilay Gai | M | Bong Liberia |
| 354. Tubman, Wilma A | F | Maryland |
| 355. Weh, Mewaseh Yah | F | Nimba Liberia |
| 356. Wullie, Kalamon | M | Lofa Liberia |
| 357. Zawolo, Jethro | M | Nimba Liberia |

**December 16, 2015**

| | | | |
|---|---|---|---|
| 358 | Ambulai, Kula Lydda | F | Cape Mount |
| 359 | Beyan, Kolu | F | Lofa Liberia |
| 360 | Blapooh, Cynthia Claress | F | Sinoe |
| 361 | Bleah, Aker Jason | M | Nimba Liberia |
| 362 | Bornguoi, George Tamba. | M | Lofa |
| 363 | Clark, Alberta J. N. | F | Lofa Liberia |
| 364 | Chineh, Romel T. | M | Maryland |
| 365 | Dargba, Best Gbain | M | Maryland |
| 366 | Dugulu, Henry Y. | M | Lofa Liberia |
| 367 | Flomo, Jonathan | M | Lofa Liberia |
| 368 | Freeman, Siedoh | F | Maryland |
| 369 | Freeman, Tabehde Princess | F | Maryland |
| 370 | Gbe, Lucretia T. | F | Grand Kru |
| 371 | Hunter, Monconjay | F | Grand Bassa |
| 372 | Jackson, Siana Tarlee | F | Bong Liberia |
| 373 | Jallah, J. Bornor | M | Lofa Liberia |
| 374 | Joe, Nyonoh Netty | F | River Cess |
| 375 | Kofa, Jr., Daniel W. | M | Sinoe Liberia |
| 376 | Kokro, Masuah T. | F | Lofa Liberia |
| 377 | Manakpalah, Charles K. | M | Nimba |
| 378 | Paye, Varbah | F | Lofa Liberia |
| 379 | Quaye, Mike Clarker | M | River Gee |
| 380 | Sankawulo, Minnie | F | Bong Liberia |
| 381 | Sanoe, Ibrahim | M | Nimba Liberia |
| 382 | Seville, II, Edwin Tegli | M | Lofa |
| 383 | Subah, Seanan O.V. | F | Lofa Liberia |
| 384 | Swaray, Issah Omaru | M | Gbarpolu |
| 385 | Tokpa, Alexander P. | M | Lofa Liberia |
| 386 | Topor, Joseph N. | M | Grand Kru |
| 387 | Udosen, Okure A. | M | Cape Mount |
| 388 | Urey, Daniel | M | Bong Liberia |
| 389 | Willicor, Alexander F. | M | Lofa Liberia |
| 390 | Woheel, Tarnue W. | M | Lofa Liberia |
| 391 | Womketeh, Joy Ngozi | F | Maryland |
| 392 | Wuoh, Arthur Jones | M | Nimba Liberia |

**December 14, 2016**

| | | | |
|---|---|---|---|
| 393. | Ajami, Ibrahim Fawzi | M | Maryland |
| 394. | Craig, II, Learwellie P. | M | Lofa Liberia |
| 395. | Duworko, Bedee S. | F | Lofa Liberia |
| 396. | Fofana, Marie | F | Montserrado |
| 397. | Garlo, Jr., J. Luke | M | Grand Bassa |
| 398. | Gbanlon, Eric G. | M | Nimba Liberia |
| 399. | Gbagornah, Peva F. | M | Lofa Liberia |
| 400. | Gbee, Jr., Emmanuel | M | Grand Kru |
| 401. | Gbollie, Elton F. | M | Lofa Liberia |
| 402. | George, Mamawah | F | Lofa Liberia |
| 403. | Hessou, Vignon Huakueh | M | Montserrado |
| 404. | Hinneh, II, Yensowah Kolobah | M | Maryland |
| 405. | Johnson, G. Galakpa | M | Lofa Liberia |
| 406. | Kabba-Kay, Melvin M. | M | Bong Liberia |
| 407. | Karnga, Dyujay Garbey | M | Grand Bassa |
| 408. | Karr, T. Juleo | M | Grand Bassa |
| 409. | Kekulah, Isaac | M | Bong Liberia |
| 410. | Kempeh, Michael Paul | M | Nimba Liberia |
| 411. | Killen, Angeline W. | F | Maryland |
| 412. | Kokolee, Gbonah W. | M | Lofa Liberia |
| 413. | Komara, Assata Sanoe | F | Nimba Liberia |
| 414. | Korkpor, Kou-Tiala Gbarpeh | F | Nimba |
| 415. | Kpaka, Jonathan Nyumah | M | Lofa |
| 416. | Krah, Amelia M | F | Grand Kru |
| 417. | Kromah, Wilhelmina Satta | F | Cape Mount |
| 418. | Lekpeh, G. Gondah | M | Nimba Liberia |
| 419. | Mahteh, Jr., Nathan Forkay | M. | Grand Kru |
| 420. | Maimie, Kpehe Jig | M | Nimba |
| 421. | Manneh, Matthew Maxwell | M | Sinoe |
| 423. | Manobah, Burgess Abraham | M | Cape Mount |
| 424. | Supuwood, Deddeh Esther Pernicia | F | Lofa |
| 424. | Tarpeh, Jewel B. | F | River Gee |
| 425. | Taylor, Emmad Saah | M | Lofa Liberia |
| 426. | Tucker, Moses Gelela | M | Bong Liberia |
| 427. | Tuopay, Rosemarie Tarneh | F | Sinoe |
| 428. | Wallace, Sr., Amelia Nyemade | F | Maryland |

| | | | |
|---|---|---|---|
| 429. | Weeks, Ruby Selma | F | Montserrado |
| 430. | Weh, Weyena | F | Bong, Liberia |
| 431. | Weidehgar, Moses U-Joe | M | Grand Bassa |
| 432. | Willie, Soeghen Emmanuel | M | Grand Bassa |
| 433. | Yarkpawolo, John Thomas | M | Lofa |
| 434. | Yeasu, Daniel Kilingsia | M | Bong |

**December 13, 2017**

| | | | |
|---|---|---|---|
| 435. | Bangbeor, Yolah F. | M | Lofa Liberia |
| 436. | Beyan, Moses K. | M | Lofa Liberia |
| 437. | Bonoe, Arnuimah G. | M | Bong Liberia |
| 438. | Coleman, Ye-Jeung G. | F | Montserrado |
| 439. | Davis, Jr., Bill Patrick. | M | Grand Bassa |
| 440. | Doe, Richard Jlah | M | Sinoe Liberia |
| 441. | Fayiah –Sam, Vickie M. N. | F | Lofa |
| 442. | Goe, Jr., Molley R. | M | Cape Mount |
| 443. | Gono, Shadrach Konan | M | Nimba Liberia |
| 444. | Gray, Alvin V. | M | Cape Mount |
| 445. | Kollie, Yarkpazuo | M | Montserrado |
| 446. | Kromah, Varmuyan A. | M | Lofa Liberia |
| 447. | Lymas, Janet S. Z. | F | Bomi Liberia |
| 448. | Mainyen, Zico W | M | Nimba Liberia |
| 449. | Odularu, Alexander O. | M | Montserrado |
| 450. | Pojah, K. Mugabe | M | Sinoe Liberia |
| 451. | Sahr, Oscar S. | M | Sinoe Liberia |
| 452. | Sando, Siaffa M. | M | Cape Mount |
| 453. | Wisseh, Clarence S. K | M | Margibi |
| 454. | Wonokay, Decontee Naa | F | Nimba Liberia |
| 455. | Wreh, J. Woyee S. | M | Grand Kru |
| 456. | Yankae, Leroy P. | M | Bong Liberia |
| 457. | Yardanmah, Luah Meshach. | M | Nimba |
| 458. | Yarngrorble, John S. | M | Bong Liberia |
| 459. | Ziah, II, Moses | M | Grand Bassa |

**December 14, 2018**

| | | | |
|---|---|---|---|
| 460 | Anandani, Tina Rajal | F | Baroda India |
| 461 | Asiedu, Kofi Nketia | M | Montserrado |

| | | | |
|---|---|---|---|
| 462 | Boduo, Tebo | M | Grand Gedeh |
| 463 | Colendo, Jesse Saah | M | Lofa Liberia |
| 464 | Darlay, Amos B.S. | M | Lofa Liberia |
| 465 | Diggs, Juliett Whyeayee | F | River Cess |
| 466 | Dukuly, Mahmoud A. | M | Lofa Liberia |
| 467 | Flomo, Jr., Anderson | M | Margibi |
| 468 | Gbozee, Johnette Gbolue | F | Lofa Liberia |
| 469 | Harris, Wilbur T.S. | M | Bong Liberia |
| 470 | Helb, Jr., James Tarnue | M | Lofa |
| 471 | Hessou, Heounohu Romello | M | Montserrado |
| 472 | Johnson, Jerome C. | M | Bomi Liberia |
| 473 | Kaba, Gassimu | M | Lofa Liberia |
| 474 | Koffeh, Amos A. | M | Lofa Liberia |
| 475 | Kolleh, Matthew | M | Bong Liberia |
| 476 | Kollie, Augustine Lear | M | Lofa Liberia |
| 477 | Kollie, James Nuakolo | M | Bong Liberia |
| 478 | Kollie, J. Ronald | M | Lofa Liberia |
| 479 | Lah, Emmanuel Dollo | M | Nimba Liberia |
| 480 | Moore, Yarvoh Massah | F | Cape Mount |
| 481 | Musa Prince C. | M | Nimba Liberia |
| 482 | Nyanfor. Mike T. | M | Maryland |
| 483 | Odoi, II, Josiah F.C. | M | Montserrado |
| 484 | Quealee, Charles G. | M | Nimba Liberia |
| 485 | Samuels, Nathaniel SunnyBoy | M | Bong |
| 486 | Sesay, Ludmila S. | F | Cape Mount |
| 487 | Sehweah, Jr., Joseph M. | M | Nimba Liberia |
| 488 | Sieh, Jr., Robert Noworway. | M | Grade Kru |
| 489 | Sieka, Theophilus | M | Grad Kru |
| 490 | Subah, Onyekachi C. | F | Lofa Liberia |
| 491 | Suberu, Adetunde Lacrown. | M | Montserrado |
| 492 | Thomas, Johnny K. | M | Nimba Liberia |
| 493 | Tyler, Dahn Henry | M | Nimba Liberia |
| 494 | Vaye, Robin | M | Nimba Liberia |
| 495 | Weah, Pauline Saeyou | F | Nimba Liberia |
| 496 | Wheh, Jr., Sylvester Oldpa | M | Grand Bassa |
| 497 | Woulu, Samson Anthony | M | Grand Kru |
| 498 | Yekeh, Tarmay Korto | F | Lofa Liberia |

| | **December 11, 2019** | | |
|---|---|---|---|
| 499 | Blamo, Romel Jeah | F | Grand Kru |
| 500 | Chea, Jestina S.H. | F | River Cess |
| 501 | Cox, Weade | F | Maryland |
| 502 | David, Emerson Garlayeedyu | M | River Cess |
| 503 | Dixon, Clarice Elena | F | Montserrado |
| 504 | Duannah, Abdoul D. | M | Lofa Liberia |
| 505 | Duru, Ben Theophilus | M | Montserrado |
| 506 | Farwenel, Ambrose | M | Lofa Liberia |
| 507 | Flomo, Emmanuel Paye. | M | Nimba Liberia |
| 508 | Gboo, Menlee | M | Nimba Liberia |
| 509 | Kanneh-Flomo, Maakah Kuo | F | Lofa |
| 510 | Kiawu, Sadatu H. | F | Cape Mount |
| 511 | Kolleh, J. Nutai | M | Bong Liberia |
| 512 | Kollie, Quoizeneh Q. | M | Lofa Liberia |
| 513 | Korpu-Miller, Hiam Marias | F | Lofa |
| 514 | Kpehe, Momo M. | M | Lofa Liberia |
| 515 | Larblah, Philip Manipaly | M | Bong Liberia |
| 516 | Luogon, Gloria C.S. | F | Montserrado |
| 517 | Mathews Sr., Roosevelt Bill | M | Grand Bassa |
| 518 | Mbayo, Moses Smart | M | Lofa Liberia |
| 519 | Mehdeh, Lawrence Dehoyusor | M. | Grand Bassa |
| 520 | Mulbah, David Dulu | M | Lofa Liberia |
| 521 | Nimley-Smith, Lydia Weahdee | F | Sinoe |
| 522 | Parker, Moses | M | Lofa Liberia |
| 523 | Paye, P. Jeffery | M | Bong Liberia |
| 524 | Peters, T. Josephus | M | Grand Bassa |
| 525 | Ricks-Dargba, Michelle | F | Montserrado |
| 526 | Sehkar, Joannis | M | Nimba Liberia |
| 527 | Smith, II, Dave Patrick | M | Grand Bassa |
| 528 | Socro, Terry Juty | M | River Gee |
| 529 | Suah, I, Maxwell Saye | M | Nimba Liberia |
| 530 | Tehoungue, Kodjo Nashapolor | M | Bong |
| 531 | Toe, Siwin Win-Win | F | River Gee |
| 532 | Weah-Weah, Korto | F | Bong Liberia |
| 533 | Wilson, Morris Yarmah. | M | Lofa Liberia |
| 534 | Yangian, Harriet | F | Nimba Liberia |
| 535 | Yiligon, Emmanuel Saye | M | Nimba Liberia |

**2020 Class: Degree Awarded March 3, 2021**

| | | | |
|---|---|---|---|
| 536. | Bartua, Josephine S.H. | F | Nimba Liberia |
| 537. | Cole, Flomo G. | M | Lofa Liberia |
| 538. | Dennis, Jr., James C. | M | Montserrado |
| 539. | Diggs, Kangar Osborne | M | Margibi Liberia |
| 540. | Freeman, Harris S. | M | Lofa Liberia |
| 541. | Garbo, Agnes Y. | F | Lofa Liberia |
| 542. | Grose, Samphina O. | F | Cape Mount |
| 543. | Gweh, Prince | M | Nimba Liberia |
| 544. | Gweama, Beyan, S. | M | Lofa Liberia |
| 545. | Jabateh, Francis Abu | M | Lofa Liberia |
| 546. | Joekolo- Ndupellar, Krystle F. | F | Nimba |
| 547. | Kamara, Alieu | M | Lofa Liberia |
| 548. | Kanneh, Morris B. | M | Lofa Liberia |
| 549. | Kpengba, Thomas T. | M | Lofa Liberia |
| 550. | Luke, Babby D. | M | Montserrado |
| 551. | Magona, Alexander S. | M | Cape Mount |
| 552. | Ndebe, Alfred M. | M | Lofa |
| 553. | Quayee Jr., Anthony S. | M | Maryland |
| 554. | Sheriff, Izetta Sianeh | F | Bong Liberia |
| 555. | Sheriff, Rukiatu M. | F | Montserrado |
| 556. | Singbe, Emmanuel T. | M | Bong Liberia |
| 557. | Tally, Seth N. | M | Grand Gedeh |
| 558. | Wiah, Yei P. | F | Nimba Liberia |
| 559. | Williams, Danma | M | Cape Mount |
| 560. | Wilson, Maerose Marina | F | Lofa Liberia |
| 561. | Wlue, Caleb Patrick | M | Maryland |
| 562. | Zwuogbae, Daanue Paye | M | Nimba |

**2021 Class: Degree Awarded March 23, 2022**

| | | | |
|---|---|---|---|
| 563. | Akinlusi-Gbolor, Priscilla M.B. | F | Montserrado |
| 564. | Cole, Aaron | M | Bong Liberia |
| 565. | Dobson, Patience Tetee | F | Grand Bassa |
| 566. | Dolopei, Deborah Ablan | F | Nimba Liberia |
| 567. | Dolopei, Jedidiah S. K. | M | Nimba Liberia |
| 568. | Eka-Tally, Eguono Josephine | F | Montserrado |
| 569. | Freeman, Motemah D. | M | Bong Liberia |
| 570. | Giddings, Diafei Frank | M | Bong Liberia |

| | | | |
|---|---|---|---|
| 571. | Gibson, Ophelia J. | F | Sinoe Liberia |
| 572. | Jerbo, Titus Bert | M | Grand Kru |
| 573. | Jusu, Jr., Saykor Ahmed. | M | Lofa |
| 574. | Kaffey, Jr., Isaac Nyenati | M | Grand Kru |
| 575. | Kamah, Avee | F | Grand Gedeh |
| 576. | Kanu, Edlyn E. | F | Margibi |
| 577. | Lamin, Hawa | F | Lofa Liberia |
| 578. | Leay, Nehwon Lovette. | F | Nimba |
| 579. | Marrah, Robert Mohammed | M | Montserrado |
| 580. | Monger, Sam Nagbe | M | Grand Bassa |
| 581. | Nyema, Milton W. | M | Grand Kru |
| 582. | Patten, Martha Racheal | F | Sinoe Liberia |
| 583. | Paye, Amos T. | M | Nimba Liberia |
| 584. | Reeves, Davidlene Anita | F | Rivercess |
| 585. | Sannoh, Varbah A. | M | Lofa Liberia |
| 586. | Snyder, S. Watchen | F | Grand Bassa |
| 587. | Sumo, Debleh O.N. | M | Gbarpolu |
| 588. | Sumo, Jr., Joseph B. | M | Lofa Liberia |
| 589. | Sumo, Famah | F | Bong Liberia |
| 590. | Siaway, Joseph Nuah | M | Nimba Liberia |
| 591. | Tah, Jr., Jacob G. | M | Grand Bassa |
| 592. | Tally, Ephraim Frake | M | Grand Gedeh |
| 593. | Tehmeh, Rogerline M. | F | Bong Liberia |
| 594. | Togbah, Adolphus Sorsor. | M | Bong |
| 595. | Tomah, Favor Lisa | F | Nimba Liberia |
| 596. | Villizu, Emmanuel J. | M | Lofa Liberia |
| 597. | Waka, Saedenu | F | Maryland |
| 598. | Walters, Ammens George. | M | Bong |
| 599. | Wegee, Jr., G. Presley Pewu. | M | Lofa |
| 600. | Yekeh, Charles D. | M | Montserrado |
| 601. | Zar, Manuel Thomas | M | Grand Bassa |
| 602. | Zarweah-Munford, Beth Z. | F | Nimba |

**SUMMARY**

**NO. OF MALES ...................426**

**NO. OF FEMALES ………….....176**

**TOTAL ................ 602**

# Appendix 4

## List of Graduates (LCPS)

### LIBERIA POSTGRADUATE COLLEGE OF PHYSICIANS AND SURGEONS (LCPS).
### LCPS Graduates (2017-2022)

**DEPARTMENT OF PEDIATRICS**

| | | |
|---|---|---|
| 1. | Dr. Cecilia Nuta | 2017 |
| 2. | Dr. Charles Oguni | 2017 |

**2018**

| | | |
|---|---|---|
| 3. | Dr. Benetta Andrews | 2018 |
| 4. | Dr. Nuntia K.Gbalon | 2018 |
| 5. | Dr. Maima Baysah | 2018 |
| 6. | Dr.Patience Franklin | 2018 |
| 7. | Dr. Hawa Sonii-Koon | 2018 |

**2019**

| | | |
|---|---|---|
| 8. | Dr. Yuah A Nemah | 2019 |
| 9. | Dr. Minnie Sankawulo-Ricks | 2019 |

**2020**

| | | |
|---|---|---|
| 10. | Dr. J Bornor Jallah | 2020 |
| 11. | Dr. G. Trokon Richards | 2020 |

**2021**

| | | |
|---|---|---|
| 12. | Dr. Joy Womketeh Cole | 2021 |
| 13. | Dr. Bedee Duworko Gbozee | 2021 |
| 14. | Dr. Melvin M. Kabba-Kay | 2021 |
| 15. | Dr. Angelne Killen | 2021 |
| 16. | Dr. Hawa Bernice Moore Kromah | 2021 |
| 17. | Dr. Wilhelmina Kromah Saydee | 2021 |

## DEPARTMENT OF INTERNAL MEDICINE

**2017**

| | | |
|---|---|---|
| 18. | Dr. Ian Wachekwa | 2017 |
| 19. | Dr. Emmanuel Ekyinabah | 2017 |
| 20. | Dr James Korvieh | 2017 |

**2018**

| | | |
|---|---|---|
| 21. | Dr. Joseph Dwana | 2018 |
| 22. | Dr. Philip Ireland | 2018 |
| 23. | Dr. Joyce Bartekwa | 2018 |
| 24. | Dr. Yassa Barclay | 2018 |

**2019**

| | | |
|---|---|---|
| 25. | Dr. Cozie Gwaikolo | 2019 |
| 26. | Dr. Tabehde Freeman-Murray | 2019 |
| 27. | Dr. Kolu Beyan Davies | 2019 |
| 28. | Dr. Varbah Paye | 2019 |

**2020**

| | | |
|---|---|---|
| 29. | Dr. Dike Christopher | 2020 |
| 30. | Dr. Nenyerker A F Vaye | 2020 |
| 31. | Dr. Lucretia Gbe-Fully | 2020 |

**2021**

| | | |
|---|---|---|
| 32. | Dr. Ibrahim F. Ajami | 2021 |
| 33. | Dr. James Luke Garlo, Jr. | 2021 |
| 34. | Dr. Eric G. Gbanlon | 2021 |
| 35. | Dr. Emmanuel W. Gbee, Jr. | 2021 |
| 36. | Dr. Isaac Kekulah | 2021 |

## DEPARTMENT OF SURGERY

**2017**

| | | |
|---|---|---|
| 37. | Dr. J Fallah Moses | 2017 |
| 38. | Dr. Solomana Konneh | 2017 |
| 39. | Dr. Terseer Utam | 2017 |
| 40. | Dr. Saygbeh Vanyanbah | 2017 |
| 41. | Dr. Torsou Jallabah | 2017 |

**2018**

42. Dr. Ansumana Camara 2018
43. Dr. Lawuoba Gbozee 2018
44. Dr. Ayun K. Cassell III 2018

**2019**

45. Dr. Kalamon Wullie 2019
46. Dr. Jonathan M. Hart 2019
47. Dr. Albertha Clarke 2019
48. Dr. Joseph Wehyee 2019

**2020**

49. Dr. Mewaseh Weh-Wesseh 2020
50. Dr. Swaliho Sheriff 2020

**2021**

51. Dr. Micheal Paul Kempeh 2021
52. Dr. Seanan O. V. Subah 2021
53. Dr. Burgess Abraham Manobah 2021
54. Dr. Soeghen Willie 2021
55. Dr. Arthur Jones Wuoh 2021

**DEPARTMENT OF OBSTETRICS/GYNECOLOGY**

**2017**

56. Dr. Paul Whessah 2017
57. Dr. Doryea Karbah 2017
58. Dr. Rosalyn Toe-Massaquoi 2017
59. Dr. Kour Geah 2017

**2018**

60. Dr. John E. Tamba 2018
61. Dr. Abraham Jawara 2018
62. Dr. Wilmot Frank 2018

**2019**

63. Dr. Kezelebah Sizi Goyah 2019
64. Dr. Korto D. Sannor 2019
65. Dr. Deazee M. Saywon 2019

66. Dr. Numeine E. Enders 2019
67. Dr. Solomon V. Harris 2019
68. Dr. Momolu Massaley 2019

**2020**

69. Dr. Henry Dugulu 2020
70. Dr. Siedoh Freeman 2020
71. Dr. Daniel Kofa 2020
72. Dr. Tarnue Woheel 2020
73. Dr. Fokape B. Duyenku 2020

**2021**

74. Dr. Best Gbain Dargba 2021
75. Dr. Weyena Weh-Gbeisay 2021
76. Dr. G. Galakpa Johnson 2021
77. Dr. Jewel Tarpeh Kollie 2021
78. Dr. Kula Ambulai-Kortimai 2021
79. Dr. Matthew M. Manneh 2021
80. Dr. Moses G. Tucker 2021

## DEPARTMENT OF FAMILY MEDICINE

**2020**

81. Dr. Patick Igwilo 2020
82. Dr. Abraham Sarnoe 2020

**2021**

83. Dr. Mamawah George-Annan 2021
84. Dr. Cynthia Claress Blapooh 2021
85. Dr. Learwellie P. Craig II 2021
86. Dr. Biligan M. Sagno-Korha 2021
87. Dr. Issah Omaru Swaray 2021

## DEPARTMENT OF OPHTHALMOLOGY

**2021**

88. Dr. George T. Bornquoi 2021
89. Dr. Unity Honey Dokie Fahn 2021

| No | Names | Year |
|---|---|---|
| **Paediatrics** | | |
| 1 | Dr. Rosemarie T. | 2022 |
| 2 | Dr. Bill Patrick Davis | 2022 |
| 3 | Dr. Chrislyn Kandakai | 2022 |
| 4 | Dr. Clarence | 2022 |
| 5 | Dr. Ruby Srelma | 2022 |
| **Internal Medicine** | | |
| 6 | Dr. Flinway Hessou | 2022 |
| 7 | Dr. Leroy P. Yankae | 2022 |
| 8 | Dr. Yensowah K. | 2022 |
| **Obstetrics/Gynecology** | | |
| 9 | Dr. Assata Komara | 2022 |
| 10 | Dr. Patience M. Martor | 2022 |
| 11 | Dr. Daniel G. Urey | 2022 |
| 12 | Dr. Alexander F. | 2022 |
| **General Surgery** | | |
| 13 | Dr. Nathan F. Mahteh | 2022 |
| 14 | Dr. Charlie M. | 2022 |
| 15 | Dr. Oscar Sahr | 2022 |
| **Psychiatry** | | |
| 16 | Dr. Moses Ziah II | 2022 |
| **Ophthalmology** | | |
| 17 | Dr. Shayri Pillai | 2022 |
| 18 | Dr. Vicky Fayiah Sam | |
| **Family Medicine** | | |
| 19 | Dr. Shadrach Konan | 2022 |
| 20 | Dr. Vignon Huakueh | 2022 |
| 21 | Dr. Masuah T. Kokro | 2022 |

# Appendix 5

## List of Deans

**A.M. Dogliotti School of Medicine College of Health Sciences 1968-2022**

| No | Names | Title | Period |
|---|---|---|---|
| 1. | Dr. Gian Carlo Setti, MD | Acting Dean | **Aug. 1, 1968 – Sept. 30, 1969** |
| 2. | Dr. Gianni Losano, MD, DIMD, Card. | Dean | **Oct. 1, 1969 – Aug. 10, 1971** |
| 3. | Dr. Luigi M. Sena, MD, D. Path. | Acting Dean | **Aug. 11, 1971 – Dec. 31, 1971** |
| 4. | Dr. Edwin M. Barclay, MD | Dean | **Jan. 1, 1972 – April 30, 1973** |
| 5. | Mrs. Agnes Cooper-Dennis, MSc. | Acting Dean | **May 1, 1973 – July 31, 1973** |
| 6. | Dr. Taiwo Daramola, BSc., MD, DPH, FMCPH | Dean | **Aug. 1, 1973 – Dec. 31, 1976** |
| 7. | Dr. Festus M. Harlay, BA, MD, FWACS | Dean | **Jan. 1, 1977 – 1983** |
| 8. | Dr. Wilmot H. Dennis, Jr., BSc, MD, OD | Acting Dean | **1984-1986** |
| 9. | Dr. Charles St. James E. Harding, MD, FRC, FWACS, MBBS | Dean | **1986 – May 1990** |
| 10. | Dr. Arthur Lewis, MSc, PhD | Acting Dean | **1992 – 1994** |
| 11. | Dr. Taiwo Daramola, BSc., MD, DPH, FMCPH | Dean | **1994 – 1996** |
| 12. | Dr. S. Benson Barh, BSc, MD, MPH, FWACP | Acting Dean | **Nov. 1, 1996 – Aug. 30, 2001** |
| 13. | Dr. Arthur Lewis, MSc, PhD | Acting Dean | **Sept. 1, 2001 – Oct. 25, 2001** |
| 14. | Dr. Tabeh L. Freeman, RN, BSc, MD, MPH, FWACP | Acting Dean | **Oct. 25, 2001 – Dec. 2010** |
| 15. | Prof. Dr. Vuyu Kanda Golakai, MD, MSc, ChM, FICS, FWACS, ScD | Dean | **January 4, 2011 to Sept. 30, 2016** |
| 13. | Dr. Z'Sherman Adams, Jr., MD, Dipl. (Cardiology) | Interim Dean | **October 1, 2016 to 2017** |
| 14. | Dr. Z'Sherman Adams, Jr., MD, Dipl. (Cardiology) | Dean | **2017 to December 2020** |
| 15. | **Dr. Lawrence M. Sherman, MD, HDS (SA), FLCS** | **Dean** | **Current** |

# Appendix 6

## Liberia Medical and Dental Council (LMDC)

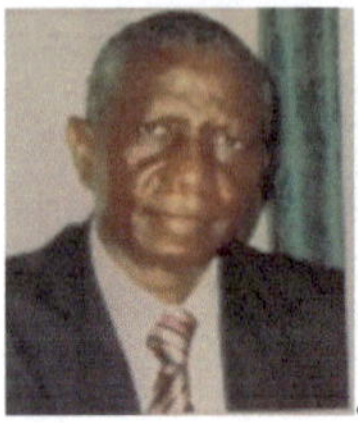

*Chairman/Prof. Robert M. Kpoto LMDC*

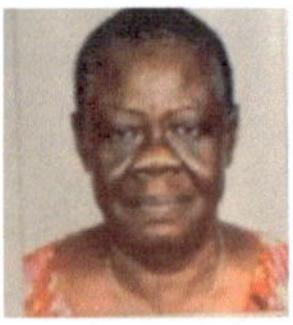

*Mrs. Cecelia Morris*

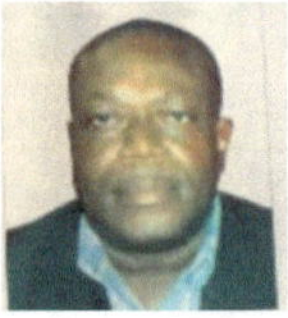

*Dr. Nyanquoi Kargbo*

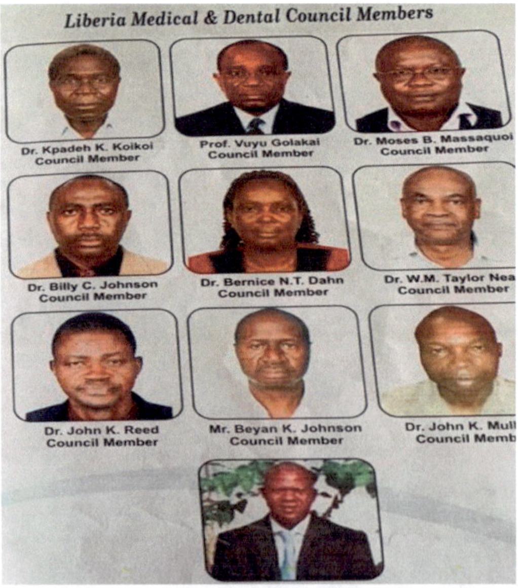

# Appendix 7

## Early Torchbearer Samuel Ford McGill

| | | | |
|---|---|---|---|
| **School** | Dartmouth Medical School | **Class** | 1839 |
| **Born** | Jan 1815, Baltimore MD | **Degree** | M.D. |
| **Died** | 21 Jun 1871, Monrovia Liberia | | |

**Career Summary**

Samuel was a Liberian Physician, Businessman and Politician. He holds a most enviable position as the first African descent to have graduated from a medical school in the United States.

**Sketch**

What is even more impressive about this achievement is that he attempting this feat when slavery was still legal in the US. The personal affront he faced, as a young man in his early twenties, from the racist system was staggering. He was a black man attempting to get an education in a time when his race was not considered equal with other races.

By the time of his graduation in 1839, he was twenty- six years old and one of the few of African descent that was in the medical profession in the world. His hard work, dedication, and persistence against nearly impossible odds is commendable. About a decade later, another African, Dr. David J. Peck, entered the medical field and in the 1860s (two decades after Dr. Mcgill became a doctor) two other Africans- Nigerian-Sierra Leoneans-, James Africanus Beale Horton and William Broughton Davies, became doctors after their training in Scotland. They also returned home to Africa.

Samuel's father, Rev. George McGill, was a Methodist lay minister. He was born a slave in1787 in Maryland, USA. He successfully purchased his freedom and that of his family. Desperate to leave the US, in 1819, he led a group of people to Haiti, but was disappointed upon arrival when he learned that the government had rescinded its earlier decision of free repatriation of peoples of color. He returned to Baltimore and eventually set sail for Liberia with his family where Samuel grew into an adolescent before he returned to America for studies.

George and his wife Angelina B. McGill had all their children in Baltimore, Maryland. They were, Samuel Ford (1813), Sarah Elizabeth (1815), James B. McGill (1817), Roszelle S. McGill (1821), and Urias Africanus McGill (1823).

**Sources:**

1. Campbell, Penelope. (Summer 1970). Medical Education for an African Colonist. *Maryland Historical Magazine*, 130-137.
2. Diemer, Andrew. (2014). The Quaker and the Colonist - Moses Sheppard, Samuel Ford McGill, and Transatlantic Antislavery across the Color Line. In Brycchan Carey & Geoffrey Plank (Eds.), *Quakers and Abolition* (pp. 135-148).
3. Champaign, IL, USA: University of Illinois Press. Champaign, IL, USA.
4. Forbush, Bliss. (1988). The Price of Freedom. *Friends Journal*, 34(9), 28-29.
5. Green, Susan. (2020). Grit and Determination. *Dartmouth Medicine* (Spring 2020). https://dartmed.dartmouth.edu/spring20/html/features_grit-and-determination/

6. Murray, Robert P. (2013). *Whiteness in Africa: Americo-Liberians and the Transformative Geographies of Race.* Ph.D., University of Kentucky.
7. Murray, Robert. (2019). Bodies in Motion: Liberian Settlers, Medicine, and Mobility in the Atlantic World. *Journal of the Early Republic* 39(4), 615-646.
8. Njoh, Joseph N. (2019). Dr. Samuel Ford McGill, M.D., and the McGill Family. In *The Beginning and Growth of Modern Medicine in Liberia and The Founding of the John F. Kennedy Medical Center, Liberia* (pp. 31-33). Nigeria: Panaf Publishing, Inc.
9. Sims, J. L., Seymour, G. L., & Anderson, B. J. K. (2003) *African-American Exploration in West Africa: Four Nineteenth-Century Diaries* (p. 370): Indiana University Press.
10. The Late Dr. McGill. (1871). *The African Repository, 47*(1), 287.

# Appendix 8

## DR. JOSEPH NAGBE TOGBA

Born December 18, 1915 in Sasstown, Dr. Togba was destined to be a physician. His uncle, a prominent traditional healer, prophesied at his birth that his nephew would be a healer like himself.

He received his primary education at the St. Paul Industrial School and then attended the College of West Africa. At seventeen in 1932, he was introduced to the practice of medicine and pharmacology at the Nana Kru Methodist Mission by Dr. Everett Veatch, an American missionary-physician from Texas.

Togba was class valedictorian at CWA, graduating in 1936. Dr. Veatch and other missionaries assisted the brilliant young student in obtaining a scholarship from the Quaker Friends College in Wichita, Kansas and he left Liberia the following year for the United States. As the first African to major in pre-med at Quaker, Togba was featured in WHO'S WHO IN AMERICAN COLLEGES AND UNIVERSITIES 1939, and graduated in 1940. He then earned his M.D. at Meharry Medical College in Nashville, Tennessee, graduating in 1944, and began nine months of residency at Homer G. Philips Hospital for "Negroes" in segregated St. Louis, Missouri. He married an American obstetric nurse, Jessye Helen Trent.

Called home in 1946 to work for the government, he was the only Liberian among 12 doctors, and assigned to the Government Hospital on Snapper Hill, which he found in disappointingly rudimentary conditions. Together with his wife, he helped establish the Nursing School, the Liberian Nurses Association, and the Liberian Board of Nurse Examiners. In the late 40s, with the assistance of the United States Public Health Service, Dr. Togba established the National Public Health System, and served as its first Director of Public Health. In 1949, he earned the MPH (Master of Public Health) from Harvard University.

Dr. Togba led the delegation to the founding conference of the World Health Organization in New York in 1948, and was appointed Secretary of Public Health RL in 1953.

At the 7th World Health Assembly conference in Geneva in 1954, he was elected president. He also served as Executive Director of the John F. Kennedy Medical Center from 1969 to 1972, and Professor and Chairman of Public Health and Preventive Medicine at the A. M. Dogliotti School of Medicine at the University of Liberia from 1972 to 1986.

Dr. Togba's personal papers were destroyed in the civil war, but fortunately he left his memoirs, published in 1993: HOW THE LORD IS MIGHTY! A DREAM IN THE JUNGLE: AUTOBIOGRAPHY OF JOSEPH NAGBE TOGBA, M.D, M.P.H.

Dr. Joseph Togba died in Silver Spring, Maryland on June 13, 2002 and remains in the ranks of the greatest practitioners of medicine produced by the Republic of Liberia, a long list that includes HENRY JENKINS ROBERTS, M.D. brother of President J.J ROBERTS, SOLOMON CARTER FULLER, M.D., JAMES SKIVRING SMITH who was also vice president of Liberia, DR. JOHN N. LEWIS JR., DR. JACOB W. PROUT, signatory to the Declaration of Independence, DR. WALTER BRUMSKINE, DR. HENRY NEHEMIAH COOPER, DR. VARSAY SIRLEAF, DR. KANDA GOLAFALE, etc. etc.

WHO Assembly President, Secretary of Public Health, RL, CMO, JFK Medical Center, Chairman, Department of Public Health, A.M. Dogliotti College of Medicine, University of Liberia.

By ***Anthony Barclay Morgan*** *Jr. for HPSOL. SOURCE: W. F. Bynum (ed.) and Belen Bynum (ed.), DICTIONARY OF MEDICAL BIOGRAPHY, 2006 Greenwood Publishing. http://www.greenwood.com/catalog/GR 2877.aspx Amos J. Beyan photo, JSTOR*

# Appendix 9

## Foundation Fellows of LCPS

**List of 55 Foundation Fellows of LCPS**

Dr. Tete K. Brooks
Dr. Tudae H. Torbor
Dr. Walter Brumskine
Dr. Walter T. Gwenigale
Dr. Willie Roberts
Prof. Joseph Njoh
Prof. Robert M. Kpoto
Prof. Vuyu Goalakai
Dr. Adams K. Lincoln
Dr. Alex Johnson
Dr. Alphonso Neemah
Dr. Angelo O. Benson
Dr. Arthur Kerkula
Dr. Benjamin Harris
Dr. Bernice T. Dahn
Dr. Billy Johnson
Dr. E. Amegashie
Dr. Edward B. Guizzie
Dr. Edward McClain
Dr. Elinor Graham
Dr. Eugene Amable
Dr. Eugene D. Dolopei
Dr. Francis N. Kateh
Dr. Ivan Camanor
Dr. J Adama Sirleaf
Dr. Jeanetta Johnson
Dr. John Mulbah
Dr. Kai Lewis
Dr. Kanda Golafalie
Dr. Laurene Whitfield
Dr. Lawrence M. Sherman
Dr. Lincoln
Dr. Mohammed Sankoh
Dr. Mohammed Sheriff
Dr. Mohammed Swaray
Dr. Moses B. F. Massaquoi
Dr. Moses Jeurolon
Dr. Moses K. Galakpai
Dr. Moses N. Pewu
Dr. Musu J. Duworko
Dr. Nathaniel S. Bartee
Dr. Peter S. Coleman
Dr. Philderald E. Pratt
Dr. Rose Macauley
Dr. Roseda E. Marshall
Dr. S. Benson Barh
Dr. Samuel Bowman
Dr. Samuel T. Dopoe
Dr. Samuel Vanii Freeman
Dr. Saye D. Baawo
Dr. Sei M. Parwon
Dr. Sia Wata Camanor
Dr. Stephen B. Kennedy
Dr. Tabeh Freeman
Dr. Tanu Duworko

# Appendix 10

## Induction Ceremony of LCPS and the Foundation Fellows

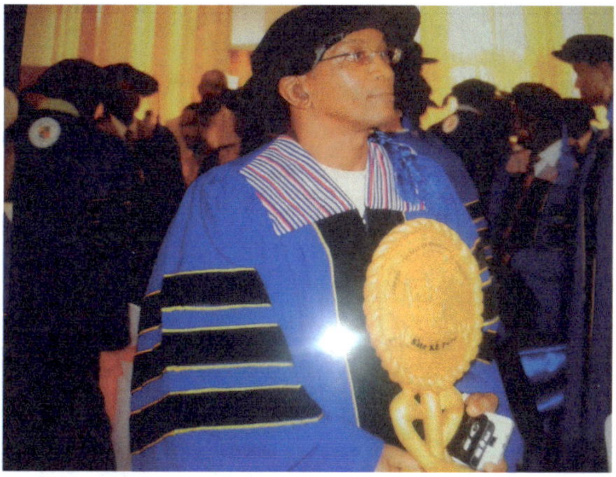

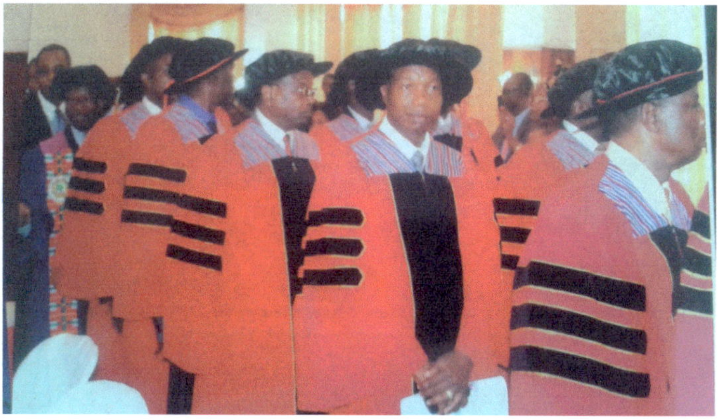

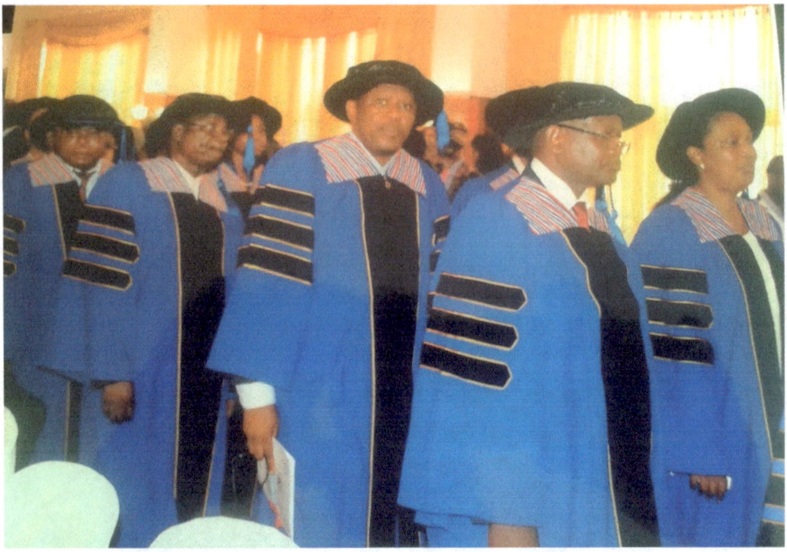

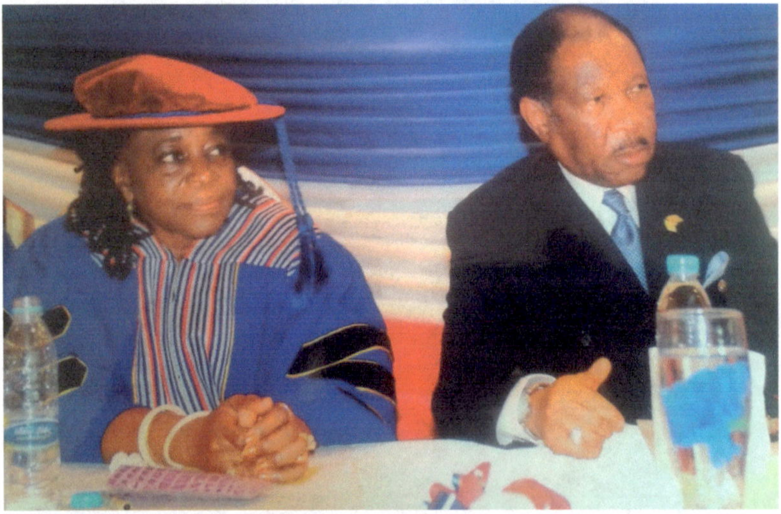

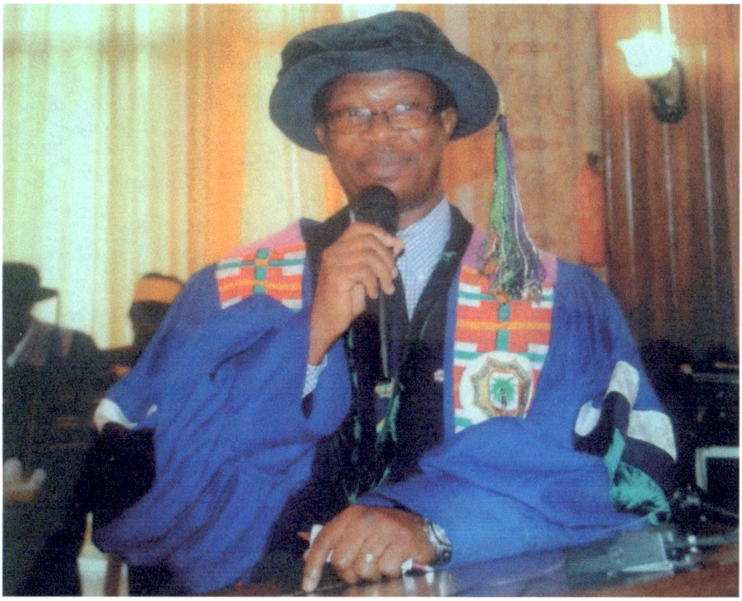

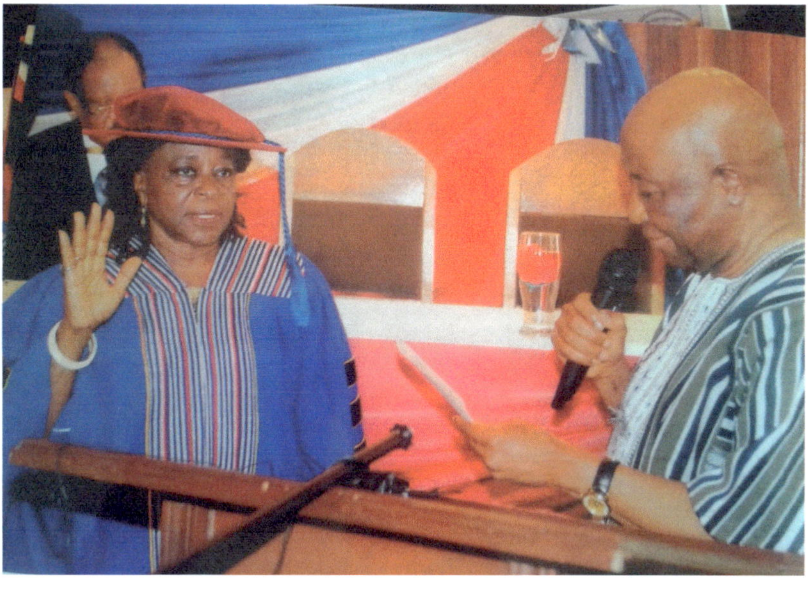

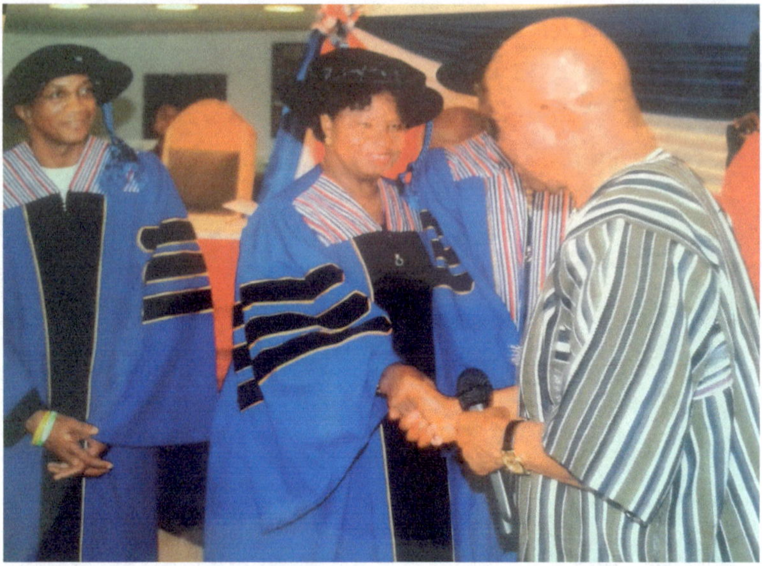

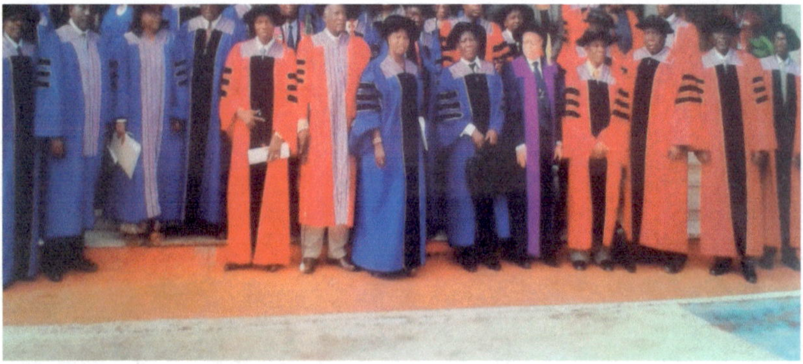

# References & Bibliography


1. Anthony B. M. Jr. for HPSOL. SOURCE: W. F. Bynum (ed.) and Belen Bynum (ed.), DICTIONARY OF MEDICAL BIOGRAPHY, 2006 Greenwood Publishing. http://www.greenwood.com/catalog/GR2877.aspx Amos J. Beyan photo, JSTOR
2. Campbell, P. (Summer 1970). Medical Education for an African Colonist. *Maryland Historical Magazine*, 130-137.
3. Diemer, A. (2014). The Quaker and the Colonist - Moses Sheppard, Samuel Ford McGill, and Transatlantic Antislavery across the Color Line. In Brycchan Carey & Geoffrey Plank (Eds.), *Quakers and Abolition* (pp. 135-148). Champaign, IL, USA: University of Illinois Press. Champaign, IL, USA.
4. Forbush, B. (1988). The Price of Freedom. *Friends Journal*, 34(9), 28-29.
5. Green, S. (2020). Grit and Determination. *Dartmouth Medicine* (Spring 2020). https://dartmed.dartmouth.edu/spring20/html/feat ures_grit-and-determination/
6. Heung, C., "Fuller, Solomon Carter (1872-1953)", *blackpast.org*
7. Keith A. P. S., (2008). *A Black Studies Primer: Heroes and Heroines of the African Diaspora,* Hansib Publications, p. 179.
8. Mohammed, H., (2021). "Recognizing African-American contributions to neurology: The role of Solomon Carter Fuller (1872–1953) in Alzheimer's disease research". *Alzheimer's & Dementia*. **17** (2): 246–250. doi:10.1002/alz.12183. ISSN 1552-5279. PMC 7986064. PMID 33325137.

9. Murray, R. (2019). Bodies in Motion: Liberian Settlers, Medicine, and Mobility in the Atlantic World. *Journal of the Early Republic* 39(4), 615-646.
10. Murray, R. P. (2013). *Whiteness in Africa: Americo-Liberians and the Transformative Geographies of Race.* Ph.D., University of Kentucky.
11. Njoh, J. N. (2019). Dr. Samuel Ford McGill, M.D., and the McGill Family. In *The Beginning and Growth of Modern Medicine in Liberia and The Founding of the John F. Kennedy Medical Center, Liberia* (pp. 31-33). Nigeria: Panaf Publishing, Inc.
12. Sims, J. L., Seymour, G. L., & Anderson, B. J. K. (2003) *African-American Exploration in West Africa: Four Nineteenth-Century Diaries* (p. 370): Indiana University Press.
13. The Late Dr. McGill. (1871). *The African Repository, 47*(1), 287.

# Index

## A



## B

## C



## D



## E

## *K*



## *L*

## *M*



## *N*



## *O*

## P



## R



## S

## T



## U



## V



## W

## *Y*



## *Z*

# About the Author

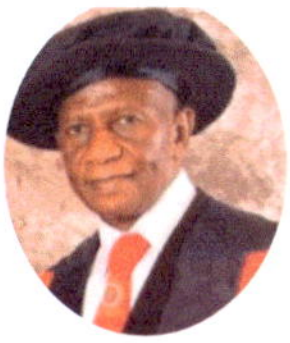

Prof. Robert Momo Zagala Kpoto is a Specialist Orthopedic Surgeon and Professor Emeritus of the A.M. Dogliotti College of Medicine (AMDCM). He is past President of the Liberia Postgraduate College of Physicians and Surgeons (LCPS); an examiner, council member, and country representative of the West African College of Surgeons (WACS).

He was born in a little village called Gellema in Lofa County unto the union of Noah (Sillah) Ziama Kpoto and Yoko Savo. Upon graduation from Junior High School, Robert came down to Monrovia to pursue higher education and graduated from medical college in 1974 as one of the Pioneer Alumini of the A. M. Dogliotti Medical College, In 1976 he departed to Europe for specialist postgraduate studies in General and Orthopedic Surgeries respectively from the University of Dublin in Ireland and the University of Liverpool in England, earning the degrees of Fellow of the Royal College of Surgeons, Ireland (FRCSI) and Masters in Orthopedic Surgery (MCh, Orth). Upon his return home in 1985 he joined the John F. Kennedy Medical Center as Consultant Orthopedic Surgeon and in 1986 promoted to Associate Professor. In 2008 he was elevated to full Professorship and head of Department of Orthopedic Surgery by Dr. Emmet Dennis President of the University of Liberia.

Professor Kpoto is a man of integrity and honesty with an unsatiable passion for cultivating the potentials and gifts of the younger generation's education through the transfer of knowledge and skills, opening of opportunities, and giving special support to the needy. His dream has been to develop and strengthen medical education and health man- power capacity of Liberia.

He considers **"THE HISTORY OF THE MEDICAL COLLEGES IN LIBERIA"** as a must be written book for the future generation. He is a Minister of the Gospel, an entrepreneur, and a philanthropist. He is married to Louise Mapleh Kpoto and they are blessed with many children.

***ALL PROCEEDS FROM SALES WILL GO INTO A TRUSTFUND TO SUPPORT THE RAFA CHILDREN'S SURGICAL HOSPITAL.***

Made in the USA
Monee, IL
05 November 2026

67808896R00105